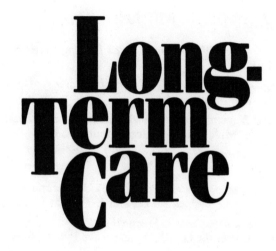

Long-Term Care

Golden Age Books
Perspective on Aging
Series Editor: Steven L. Mitchell

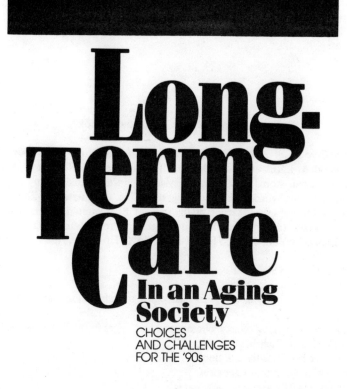

Long-Term Care

In an Aging Society

CHOICES
AND CHALLENGES
FOR THE '90s

Gerald A. Larue and Rich Bayly

Golden Age Books

Prometheus Books • Buffalo, New York

Published 1992 by Prometheus Books

96 95 94 93 92   5 4 3 2 1

Library of Congress Cataloging-in-Publication Data

Long-term care in an aging society: choices and challenges in the '90s / [edited] by Gerald A. Larue and Rich Bayly.
        p.   cm.—(Golden age books)
    Includes bibliographical references
    ISBN 0-87975-712-4 (paper : alk. paper)
    ISBN 0-87975-695-0 (cloth : alk. paper)
    1. Aged—Long term care—United States. I. Larue, Gerald A. II. Bayly, Rich.
III. Series.
HV1461.L66   1992
362.6'0973—dc20   91-18979
                                                                          CIP

Printed in the United States of America on acid-free paper.

Preface

This collection was prompted by a successful national conference held in Calgary, Alberta, June 3–6, 1990. Each year, the Canadian Long-Term Care Association (CLS) sponsors a national conference in Canada, and in 1990 the Alberta Long-Term Care Association (ALTCA) hosted the event.

We decided on a policy-oriented event to start the decade of the nineties. We wanted health-care CEOs, legislators, policy planners, and consumer advocates to meet together with leaders in the industry. The intent was to create a clearer, consistent vision of the choices facing long-term care decision-makers in the decade ahead. The search for topics and speakers brought together individuals who expressed their views forcefully and with appreciation for the level of commitment and cooperation required to achieve progress.

Throughout the three-day conference, we witnessed a build-up of emotion and intensity that led to standing ovations and to presentations that brought the audience to tears. This outcome was never anticipated, particularly in a crowd of over five hundred seasoned experts who shape, run, and use Canada's long-term care system.

It is increasingly clear that a broader range of individuals must understand the pressures facing our aging society. It is our hope that this publication will help in the making of better choices in long-term care during the coming decade of change.

Rich Bayly
Alberta Long-Term Care Association

Contents

8   Contents

Introduction

Long-term care for elders has become a pressing issue for families, communities, and governments at every level. During the past century some twenty-eight years have been added to life expectancy, and with increased longevity have come dramatic shifts in life patterns. Elders move from independence to semi-independence to what in some cases is full dependency. Health care has thus become a pressing social problem. Canada has a national health-care program that embraces all citizens from cradle to grave; is devoid of red tape; and, as our contributors to this volume note with some apprehension, is faced with mounting costs. No such program exists in the United States, where Medicare and Medicaid programs are cluttered with administrative paperwork and some citizens become poverty stricken in their attempt to meet the rising costs of health care. Here, too, long-term costs are a major issue. At the same time, each of our writers recognizes the importance of personal dignity and self-control over life as elders become dependent on others for care and on governmental assistance for support.

As Rich Bayly has noted, this volume provides a look at long-term care in the decade ahead. A group of distinguished health-care advocates have been assembled to offer their valuable insights into the choices and challenges facing caregivers (whether professional or nonprofessional), families, long-term care institutions, and government agencies. It was clear that these perspectives had to be shared with a larger audience.

9

On my return to the United States, I talked with researchers and scholars at the University of Southern California's Andrus Center about the issues raised in Calgary. Two chapters were added in an effort to broaden the volume's scope by including two distinctly American perspectives. Linda A. Wray and Fernando M. Torres-Gil introduce problems encountered on the American scene, particularly in California. Kathleen H. Wilbur and Leah Buturain present one of the emerging services in long-term care, namely, money management for the elderly.

I had met Eva Skinner earlier at an Andrus Center meeting on ethical issues in aging. Her clear grasp of major concerns prompted an invitation to contribute to this volume. Her chapter on long-term care as *the* women's issue for the coming decade draws attention to the fact that women bear the greatest responsibility in this demanding field. Mary Ann Barnhart, who works with problem elders whose behavior significantly challenges caretakers, draws our attention to one of the most demanding services of long-term care.

In December, 1991, the Alberta Council on Aging, the Alberta Association on Gerontology, the Centre for Gerontology, and the Alberta Long-Term Care Association sponsored a Conference in Edmonton, Alberta, titled "The Dawn of a New Age." Rich Bayly and I were both involved—he as an organizer and I as a coordinator. One of the most important contributors to the Conference was the Honorable Monique Vézina, minister of state for seniors and the spokesperson for seniors in the Canadian cabinet. She has graciously granted us permission to publish her address as the opening chapter of this book.

It must be noted that there are obvious differences in style among the chapters. The Canadian conference papers were, for the most part, prepared primarily for a listening audience. Though many of the personal asides, intimate anecdotes, and political remarks have been eliminated, something of the warm informality of the spoken presentations does remain.

The contributors do not pretend to provide final answers to the problems they consider. Their comments are intended to invite thoughtful commentary and dialogue in pertinent facets of long-term care as we look ahead to a new millennium.

The editors express their grateful appreciation for the help of Anna Ball, Administrative Assistant, Alberta Long-Term Care Association. Her warm personality and cheerful acceptance of responsibilities associated with the transcription of taped materials lightened our editorial responsibilities. Steven L. Mitchell, editor of Prometheus Books's Golden Age series, a trusted friend of long standing, has been both patient and understanding with delays. As always, Paul Kurtz, editor-in-chief of Prometheus Books, has been supportive and encouraging.

Gerald A. Larue
Andrus Center
University of Southern California

1

Are We Ready to Meet the Challenge?

The Honorable Monique Vézina

"The kind of life older people in our society can live is the kind of life we will live. For this reason alone aging ought to be of concern to us all."

V. Marshall, 1980

In 1991, virtually everyone knows that the aging of the population will be one of the most significant social phenomena in the next few decades. Statistics on this are coming at us from all sides. Studies are constantly appearing, but my impression is that, unfortunately, there is still more talk than action. In the minds of all too many Canadians—and this includes too many politicians—the aging of our population is set aside in a pigeonhole for "dealing with later."

To consider the aging of our population as a problem that needs to be resolved is, in my mind, an error, a view that is harmful from a number of different perspectives. First of all, it places aging in competition with other political and economic challenges we must all face at this time. The result is that we do not respond to the challenge of our aging population. In the current context, it is not being given the same importance as other issues, such as national unity, global competition, unemployment, and so on. This is why we "put off until tomorrow" what we could and perhaps should be doing today.

But, it is on a much more fundamental level that viewing our aging population as a "problem to be resolved" is harmful. In fact, aging is *not a problem* but a reality, which we, as a society, must face and plan for. In the not-too-distant future seniors will represent close to 20 percent of the Canadian population. Then our society will be quite different from what it is today.

I must admit that we are at least talking more about aging than we did just a few years ago. As well, I see seniors asserting themselves more and more. But it seems to me that these changes are occurring within a climate of some indifference, and that indifference must be questioned, given the time-frame within which we have to react.

The year 2000 is just around the corner. We can, of course, prepare bit by bit, looking at today's situation in the light of demographic projections. But there is another option, one that I consider far preferable. This is to promote and to generate today a vision of tomorrow's society, an older society, a society in which all of its members can develop their full potential.

We need, however, to develop an accurate view of just what aging is. I feel that too many people still believe in the myths about aging, and so we must promote realistic images of older Canadians. Aging is a natural process and is too often associated with disease. I am concerned about the consequences of such false perceptions.

One would hope that by the turn of the century seniors will be regarded as an important resource to society. You will, I hope, agree with me that, in a world preoccupied with preserving the environment and making the best use of resources, it would be unacceptable to waste the wealth of experience and knowledge of our seniors.

While we have seen some improvements in the response to seniors' concerns, much still remains to be done. We must continue with increased effort if we wish to make sure that society knows and understands those who will soon make up a quarter of its population.

Over the past three years, I have noted that other myths and stereotypes exist which affect people's perception of seniors. One, which is still far too common, is the misconception that all seniors are alike. I have met thousands of seniors in the past few years. I can state that the evidence they have provided to me is of their vast diversity, not their homogeneity.

I have also come to realize that we are committing an error if we consider chronological age as the only measure of someone's capacity to function independently. To examine the impact of an aging society with any degree of accuracy, it is more important to look at factors relating to autonomy.

When the prime minister entrusted me with my mandate for seniors, I sometimes heard talk of the "third age," the "fourth age," and sometimes even the "fifth age." I will admit that I was not very receptive to these concepts. I found that they complicated things greatly and placed us at risk of limiting the debate on aging only to the "experts." Today, I am just as resistant to labelling and to verbal "overkill," which tends only to mystify people.

It is worth keeping in mind that 90 percent of people over the age of sixty-five live quite independently in the community outside of an institution. We need to take note of all those people aged sixty-five, seventy, seventy-five, and often eighty or more who are keeping active, exercising, getting involved, and meetng challenges.

I am convinced that independence will be a key factor in the organization of an aging society. I also believe that we shall have to *promote it, encourage it, and respect it.* We must recognize the need to help others, and accept help ourselves.

The concepts of third and fourth age may seem to be a great invention of and for the experts, but it does reflect a reality: that the criterion of autonomy must be considered before chronological age in recognizing full participation in the socio-economic life of a country. Looking toward tomorrow without a clear awareness of this reality is an error in judgment.

Since we must start right away to look toward tomorrow, the young and the not so young, the politicians and all citizens, must rid themselves of these false perceptions about aging and learn instead to consider the full potential of older people in society. I don't see this as meaning that we must contest people's right to retire but that we must assess with accuracy and realism the needs and expectations of an older society. Then we must consider all of the ways to meet those needs and expectations using *all of the available resources.*

I believe in the solidarity of our society, and the importance of the contribution of *all of its resources* to reach our shared objectives. Building the Canadian society of the next century requires us to acknowledge seniors' ability to meet challenges and to fulfill a socioeconomic role.

Some of you may suspect that I am about to propose doing away with retirement! I don't know whether you will find this reassuring, but I must tell you that I have both positive and negative feelings about retirement. In fact, I fear that association between "retirement from work" and "retirement from life." I believe that individuals deserve the right to retire from working. However, withdrawal from society would be harmful for them and for the rest of us.

There is a fairly broad social consensus that age sixty-five is "the age of retirement." This is no longer completely true; nevertheless, the majority of people do take retirement from work between the ages of sixty and sixty-five. This situation will probably continue to evolve over the next few years. Some seniors now choose to maintain or reestablish connections with the workplace, through job-sharing, contract work, or placement agencies. Those who do, appreciate the opportunity to use their skills but at a pace that suits them better. Their employers also benefit from their availability, their expertise, and their reliability. This is why I support the *right* to retire from work but not enforced retirement. This seems to me to be more in line with the flexibility required by an aging society.

In our first national strategy aimed at seniors, we created the seniors independence program, which illustrates the effectiveness of the dynamism and socioeconomic potential of seniors. This program for seniors funds projects that empower seniors. Senior autonomy is in itself a great resource for the community. By encouraging it, we improve seniors' quality of life. It must also be acknowledged that independence encourages activity, and that activity itself enriches the socioeconomic assets of a country.

There is, however, still too much of a tendency to take this involvement by seniors lightly. I have the impression that, in general, it is seen as letting them do what they want because it is a good thing to keep them occupied. But such an attitude does not recognize the value of their involvement in the day-to-day functioning of our communities. Not only is the contribution of seniors not recognized, but all too often our reaction implies that seniors' work is not essential for the efficient functioning of our society. Such a reaction strikes me as regrettable, and potentially unhealthy as our society is transformed by the phenomenon of aging.

Seniors have vast potential. For the most part they have retired from the work force, but they have not retired from society. Not only must their participation be welcomed, but they must also have expectations placed on them—expectations that, while being reasonable and realistic are also concrete and self-actualizing. Society has a right to benefit from their experience. I cannot see how we can build a solid society if we leave a quarter of our population on the sidelines. This would be a blatant waste of human potential.

I feel that we must free ourselves of the discomfort we feel at reexamining our concept of retirement. Personally, I would like to see us confirm that retirement from a job is a right, but I would also like to see us have the courage to tell seniors that society needs them to attain the common social goal of well-being for all. Our future lies in being frank with seniors in the message we send out.

We need to acknowledge seniors' status and their socioeconomic role so that they will be fully involved in the changes our society will undergo.

What I want to see, above all else, is that we cease to look at aging only in the context of theoretical studies, of interest primarily to researchers. My reflection, inspired by experience in politics and three years as the minister responsible for seniors, leads me to the conclusion that the time is ripe for us to move forward in our thinking.

In recent years, Canadian seniors have made themselves heard and their influence felt (much more than their counterparts in some European countries). We need to encourage this assertiveness.

Starting at this very moment, we must begin to raise the consciousness of all generations in our society about the reality of aging. We must all be part of planning for an older society, one that will be dynamic and respectful of the needs and aspirations of all its members. We must therefore make sure that we go further—that we begin to *face the future together*— with the seniors of today and tomorrow. I am convinced that no one is better placed to begin this process than the seniors of today. Their lucidity, wisdom, common sense, and social responsibility provide them with everything needed to assume leadership in a debate on the organization of tomorrow's society—the society of our children and grandchildren.

2

Health-Care Policy

Michael Rachlis

What choices do people really have? Here is a scenario that is far too common. Mr. Smith, sixty-five years old, has just retired. He finds he is not sleeping well. Since he is around the house all the time, he gets on his wife's nerves; they're not getting on well together. They go to a shopping mall one day, and as they pass a walk-in clinic Mrs. Smith says, "You've been complaining for a couple of weeks about not sleeping well at night. Why don't you go in and see the doctor?"

The physician prescribes a valium-type drug and tells Mr. Smith to see his family physician for follow-up. Unfortunately, what often happens in medical care is that once a prescription is written, it is engraved in stone. The family doctor continues the medication. The drug, sold as a sleeping medication, unfortunately, stays in the body twenty-four hours and can impair performance during the day. So, about six months later, during the winter, Mr. Smith, who is by this time slightly impaired from the medication he has been taking for sleep, falls and breaks his ankle and is admitted to the hospital for surgery.

We pick up Mr. Smith about five years later at age seventy. He has now developed some arthritis. The pain is mild but it's enough to warn him when the weather is going to change. He goes to his doctor, complains of the pain, and learns that he appears to have osteoarthritis. A nonsteroidal anti-inflammatory (aspirin-like) drug is prescribed. This medi-

19

cation is safer than aspirin in that it causes less frequent gastrointestinal (GI) bleeding than aspirin, but it certainly is not risk free. About two months later, Mr. Smith has a GI bleed and is admitted to the hospital in need of acute care.

He recovers. Three years later, at age seventy-three, he develops chest pains as he shovels snow. After a few tests, his doctor recommends that he have bypass surgery. Unfortunately, while on the operating table he has a rather serious stroke, with persistent hemiplegia* and some dys-phasia.† When Mr. Smith gets out of the hospital, he deteriorates. Mr. and Mrs. Smith get assistance from their one daughter but Mr. Smith now requires so much care that they are really at their wits' end. They arrange for home care but unfortunately it isn't available in the evenings or on the weekends when Mr. Smith is at his worst. Finally, his daughter, who has moved in with him at great cost to her family life, quickly experiences emotional burn-out and suffers a psychological breakdown. Consequently, Mr. Smith is admitted to an acute care facility. He remains there, despite the fact that he undergoes no medical treatment. After four months he is discharged to a nursing home.

In the nursing home Mr. Smith continues to deteriorate. Both his daughter and his wife visit, but his daughter has grown discouraged about the whole situation. Mr. Smith continues to deteriorate and is eventu-ally admitted to an acute care hospital where he is treated for pneumonia. He now requires such intensive care that the nursing home feels it can no longer accommodate him. He remains in the acute care hospital for six months. He is next discharged to a chronic care hospital and, several years later, at the age of seventy-eight, Mr. Smith dies of a massive stroke.

I'd like to recast that scenario, in a future setting representing the way I hope it might be by the time I'm Mr. Smith's age. Personal choices, for patients and their families, are fundamental in a long-term health care system. The need for patient choice has been highlighted in a number of reports and commissions during the last few years, such as the 1987 Ontario Health Review Panel chaired by Doctor John Evans. Their pri-mary recommendation was to give patients more informed choices about their care. The Rochon Commission report, which, in my estimation, is the finest report on health care that has come out of Canada in the last five years, also highlighted, as one of its major points, that individuals (for all the platitudes we mouth about informed consent) are not offered

---

*paralysis of one side of the body
†lack of coordinated speech and/or failure to arrange one's words in an understand-able way

proper choices to guide their own care. So what would a health-care system that offered real choices look like?

Let's start over again. At the age of sixty-five, Mr. Smith can't go to a walk-in clinic. There are none. But government policies have encouraged and required the development of comprehensive primary care centers. Therefore he can contact the health-care system through his regular means of care without an undue wait. He goes to his family doctor, who isn't paid primarily on a fee-for-service basis, and therefore is not financially penalized by seeing only three to four patients per hour. The doctor diagnoses that Mr. Smith's sleep disturbance is related to his recent retirement. (Of course the ideal scenario in our health and social services system should include comprehensive pre-retirement planning, but then there would be very little to this story.) The doctor spends a much longer time on a second interview with Mr. Smith and his wife.

The doctor refers Mr. Smith to the health center's social worker. This health center is staffed not just by doctors but by nurses, nurse practitioners, social workers, rehabilitation staff and others. The social worker counsels Mr. Smith and his wife. The clinic worker learns that Mr. Smith has always enjoyed woodworking as a hobby. The social worker knows that the local community center, which offers an after-school program for children, is looking for volunteers for their crafts program. She refers Mr. Smith to the program.

As a result of being active and feeling useful again, Mr. Smith does not need to take any sleeping medication and he no longer breaks his ankle. Five years later, however, he does develop mild osteoarthritis because he has had a previous injury to that ankle. He goes to his doctor, who diagnoses the condition and despite the drug company information that everyone with osteoarthritis needs a nonsteroidal anti-inflammatory drug, the doctor offers Mr. Smith a choice. He could opt for physical therapy when the ankle acts up, stay off it for a while, apply heat, and when the ankle is feeling well—which is most of the time—he could engage in muscle-strengthening exercises. If medication is warranted, Mr. Smith could take some acetaminophen (e.g., Tylenol®), a drug similar to aspirin but with virtually no GI upset. On the days he doesn't have any pain, he takes no tablets. Conversely, more tablets can be taken on the days when he does have pain. Or he can take a nonsteroidal anti-inflammatory drug on an as-needed basis. After all the discussion, Mr. Smith chooses to try to strengthen the ankle and use the tylenol as needed. As a result, the subsequent GI hemorrhage is averted and the acute care is not required for that episode.

At age seventy-six, Mr. Smith develops angina, but now it doesn't develop until he's three years older because he's had decreased mental stress in his life. It is well documented that mental stress can lead to angina. He does undergo a diagnostic workup, however, and is found to have what is called triple vessel disease, but instead of a recommendation for bypass surgery his doctor now explains the situation as follows:

There is evidence that bypass surgery may increase life expectancy for people with this problem; however, the experimental studies of bypass surgery have not included any elderly patients. In fact, only one study included patients up to the age of seventy; all the other studies have excluded subjects older than sixty-five. The average age for patients in these studies was the early fifties. Therefore the doctor cautions Mr. and Mrs. Smith that the results of these studies may not apply to an older population. The doctor also mentions that bypass surgery is not like an appendectomy, in which there is about a 100 percent chance of survival if it is removed and no chance of survival if it isn't. While there is a statistical improvement of life expectancy of about one to three percent per year, ominously, the stroke rate for patients in their seventies, following bypass surgery, is about eight times higher than it is for patients in their fifties.

With this information, the Smiths decide not to go ahead with bypass surgery. Mr. Smith is advised that quitting smoking is as effective an intervention in improving his life expectancy as having bypass surgery. So he quits smoking. He also increases his exercise in a closely monitored fashion, and because of the osteoarthritis in his ankle, he takes up swimming, after discussion with his rehabilitation therapist at the clinic.

We can't say that death is ever something that is avoided entirely. The iron law of epidemiology is that everybody dies. However, instead of having his stroke at the age of seventy-three while having bypass surgery, Mr. Smith now has a stroke at the age of eighty. When he comes to the emergency department of his local hospital, instead of being admitted, he and his wife are met by a quick response team, similar to the one that's been developed for the Victoria Health Project, one of the most exciting projects in the country. So Mr. Smith is sent home. He's never admitted to the hospital in the first place and he receives full rehabilitation—physical, psychological, and social—and his family is fully involved in his rehabilitation.

Of course he does deteriorate over time, but every step of the way he's followed actively by his family doctor, the nurses at the health center, and by his social worker. Over time, his wife and daughter need more and more support to care for him. So initially he starts going to a day program once a week. Then he starts using it more. Respite care becomes involved to spell the family and allow them a few breaks during the week. All of this provides added flexibility. Now, Mr. Smith might take eight

Tylenol® tablets a day when he's having more pain, four when the pain is mild, and none when he doesn't need them at all. Eventually he does die, but he dies at home during his sleep with his family around him. For me that's the system I hope we will have in place by the time I need long-term care.

The reform of Canada's long-term care system is intimately intertwined with reform of the health-care system as a whole. But what's wrong with Canada's health-care system and how might we go about trying to fix it? First, the health-care system is not the major determinant of our health. One of the great illusions in the twentieth century is that the doctor and hospital care are what make us healthy. During the twentieth century there have been tremendous increases in life expectancy. Canadians in 1990 are some of the healthiest human beings who have ever lived in the million years that human beings have walked the planet. We've poured hundreds of billions of dollars into our health care system and we've come to believe in a direct cause and effect relationship, that doctors and hospital care have made us healthy. But that's not the case.

If we look at the infectious diseases, which were the scourges of the nineteenth century, almost without exception by the time there was an effective medical intervention (antibiotic or a vaccine) available to treat or prevent them, the mortality from these diseases had already been slashed. The best example would be tuberculosis. In 1900 it was the number-one killer in North America and there wasn't an effective intervention developed against it until 1948 when the antibiotic streptomycin became widely available. The sanatoriums probably did do some good by enabling patients to gain strength to fight the disease. Looking back, the impact of that service was minimal; what really made the difference between 1900 and 1948, when 90 percent of the mortality from TB was eliminated, was improved social and economic conditions. By the time streptomycin became available, tuberculosis had been almost wiped out.

I'm not suggesting that we should throw out the baby with the bathwater. I don't want to get rid of what's good about our system. I want to preserve it. But I think we need to recognize that it isn't acute medical care and hospital care that has made the big difference in life expectancy in this century. The analysis of TB holds for virtually every other infectious disease: cholera, measles, scarlet fever, and so on. There are some exceptions. For polio we did need the vaccine before we could deal effectively with that disease.

Faced with heart disease and cancer as our major killers, many still assume that we must rely on medical research and medical care to deal with these physical conditions. First, regarding heart disease: In Canada during the last thirty years, the death rates from heart disease have fallen over 30 percent. In fact, they are now falling at a rate of about 30 percent per year, which means that by the year 2000 we are going to be about two-thirds less likely to die of heart disease than we were in the sixties. This has been a remarkable achievement, almost paralleling the way that TB declined in the first few decades of this century. But why has this happened? Although it is difficult to agree on the exact numbers, I have not read a scientific paper suggesting that a majority of the decline was due to medical care. All the analyses conclude that at least 60 percent of the decline in deaths due to heart disease is the result of decreased cholesterol levels, decreased smoking in the population, improved exercise, and other social factors. So it's not by and large medical care that has been responsible for the tremendous achievement of decreasing the rates of heart disease death in our country.

What about cancer? People tend to believe that we're winning the war against cancer because that's what we've been told for a number of years. But we're not winning. We are about 5 to 10 percent more likely to die from cancer at every age in this country now than we were just thirty to thirty-five years ago. Why is this happening? There have been major advances in the medical treatment of some cancers, such as childhood leukemia and Hodgkins disease. On the other hand, if we look at the major cancers that claim so many victims—breast cancer, bowel cancer, lung cancer—medical care has not made much impact on these. The age-adjusted death rates from lung cancer have gone through the roof. The death rates for lung cancer in women have gone up 400 percent in the last twenty years. We're not talking about a disease that affects small numbers of people. Thousands die from lung cancer. This is an epidemic of mass proportions, and the rising rate of lung cancer is the reason we're losing the war against cancer. The good news is that we can deal with this epidemic. We know that we can virtually eliminate cigarette smoking in a generation if we have the political will to do so through banning all cigarette promotions, through making all public spaces nonsmoking, and so on. If we're going to deal with heart disease and cancer, it will be in much the same way we dealt with TB in the first decade of this century—by improving social and economic conditions. That's what's going to make the difference in improving the health of our country. I'm not throwing out medical care, but the more we focus on medical care, the further away we get from solving the real problems that result in disease.

The second guide to health-care reform is awareness of the fact that the health-care system is not nearly as efficient as we like to believe it is. We like to believe that our health-care system operates at the cutting edge of efficiency, but many of us within the system know that's not true.

We Canadians overuse institutions tremendously. We have high rates of acute-care hospitalization and we also have a lot of elderly people living their lives in institutions. Canada has one of the highest rates of institutionalizaton of its elderly of any nation in the world. The answer to the problem of chronic-care patients in acute-care settings is clearly not to build more chronic-care beds but to make more efficient use of existing personnel. Research indicates that specially trained nurses could do at least one-half the work of general practitioners, as well or better. The reason to use nurses and other health-care professionals instead of physicians, is not primarily to save money, although that's laudable in itself, but because by and large they will do those jobs better than physicians and their services are far less expensive.

The next guide to long-term health-care reform is related to the use of drugs. The overuse of prescription medications in Canada is a scandal. The real problem in this country is not illegal drugs on the school grounds but the poisoning of seniors with medications prescribed by doctors and paid for out of the public purse by drug programs.

Some studies suggest that 20 percent of senior admissions to institutions were directly caused by adverse reactions to prescription drugs. I think that's a high figure. But even if you took about 2 percent or so, which would be about the lowest that the literature would indicate, Canadians are looking at a cost of hundreds of millions of dollars in acute hospital care. And we're looking at perhaps half a billion dollars of unnecessary and therefore potentially dangerous drugs being prescribed for seniors every year, all of which is paid for with public funds. Altogether at least a billion dollars is not doing us any good. Why does this happen?

Only someone outside the health-care system can think logically about all this, because those of us within the system are unable to deal with it. In medical school or postgraduate training, doctors receive very little training in the proper prescribing of drugs. When they eventually start their own practice, doctors are wooed by drug companies who spend somewhere between four and six thousand dollars per doctor to try to convince physicians to prescribe their products.

Like any expert marketers, drug companies rely on focus groups (small groups of about five doctors) to find out how to market their drugs properly. They bring the doctors in and tell them they are going to be helpful in developing new products. Actually, the drug companies seek to uncover points of resistance to prescribing a particular product the company is thinking of marketing. In fact, that's one of the reasons thalidomide was prescribed as a sedative for pregnant women—not because it was safe—but when the marketers were doing their study they found out physicians were looking for a safe sedative for pregnant women, so they marketed thalidomide from that angle. The focus group found that the physicians' point of resistance was concern about the safety of certain drugs for pregnant women. When drug companies have that much world-wide expertise, marketing plans that work in one geographic area are instantly transferred to another. We know that many thousands of dollars are spent per capita to try to convince doctors to prescribe one product, but how much energy, money, and resources do federal and provincial governments, colleges, and physicians' groups spend to try to make sure that doctors prescribe properly? It can't be more than about one hundred dollars per physician. Then the material that you do get from government agencies or a medical organization tends to have lots of small print rather than the glossy pictures and big print of the drug company advertisements. This is a problem of scandalous proportions. Some geriatricians say that government and our colleges of physicians and surgeons, and to a certain extent our colleges of pharmacy, are permitting the prescription drug problem to kill thousands of Canadians every year. Even if the number was just hundreds, that's far more than the number of deaths due to illegal drugs every year in this country. This accounts for a billion dollars a year that is not available to other areas of health care, including long-term care.

Excessive testing represents another area where there is waste in our system. There is far too much testing of prospective medications. Most elderly people are healthy, but because older persons have chronic illness, they are subject to more medical intervention of all sorts including diagnostic tests. Add to this the fact that we are over-producing physicians. The population of physicians in Canada is growing at about 3.5 to 4 percent per year while the national population is growing at only 1 percent per year. The costs of medical care are directly related to the number of doctors.

How can we develop a reformed health policy? First, we need to set goals for health based on a vision of health and fundamental social values. Second, we need to use the best available research information to plan a strategy for achieving these goals. Third, health promotion and the health-care system are the two main concerns in a strategy for improved health. Fourth, healthy public policy is the most important component of a health promotion program. By healthy public policy I mean legislative action against cigarette smoking as well as getting doctors and other health-care workers to counsel their patients against smoking.

Finally, in the cruelest single act of any government in this country in the last twenty years, in an attempt to cut our deficit to tens of billions of dollars, the federal government cut 1.6 million dollars from women's programs, 1.2 million of which went to funding eight women's centers throughout the country particularly in rural areas of Quebec and Atlantic

Canada. The fact that eighty such centers could be funded for 1.2 million is astounding. Why something so efficient is closed down is beyond my imagining. In many communities these were the only resources for women in abusive relationships. Each year in Canada between fifty and a hundred women lost their lives at the hands of spouses or lovers through acts of violence, and this represents a major health problem in our country. Again, money and lives are in conflict.

How do governments decide what programs they're going to fund? Ultimately they must look at setting some sort of goals for health. We've been guided in our program development in Canada by a fascination with bricks and mortars rather than with concern for the ultimate health of the population. However, all that's going to be changing very shortly. In reforming health care, we first have to allow patients to make informed choices and let this guide the demand for resource allocation. Second, we have to decentralize and democratize the decision making about resource allocation and planning, and that means more regionalization of health care. Third, we need to implement real quality assurance mechanisms because Canada lacks so much quality assurance in its health-care system. We have focused on structure and process with the lack of attention to outcomes. Had we run our grain industry, fishing industry, lumber industry, or auto industry with the quality assurance we have in our health-care system, we would have gone broke years ago. Fourth, we need to change the financial incentives for health care.

I'd like to give an example of the type of program we're considering that would meet some of these criteria. This is the On Lok Seniors program in San Francisco. The On Lok Senior Health Services opened its nonprofit operation for the frail elderly in 1973. Today there are three day centers in the north beach area of San Francisco through which three hundred very high-risk clients are served. The average age of these clients is the early eighties and they have five or six serious medical diagnoses each. Many are very frail, three-quarters are incontinent, a similar number have difficulty using their limbs, and many are at special risk because of poverty and isolation. Two-thirds of the participants live alone and two-fifths are poor enough to qualify for supplemental security income. Most participants are from the Chinese community but there are people from Philippino and Italian communities as well as blacks and Caucasians. To participate in the program, the applicants must be over fifty-five and medically assessed by a state representative as needing nursing home care. But instead of becoming institutionalized, On Lok enrollees remain in their own familiar surroundings and receive whatever support they require to remain there. In that way, On Lok is not totally dissimilar from the assessment process that goes on in some of our Canadian Provinces. The participants who qualify for both Medicare and Medicaid pay nothing. In the United States Medicare pays institutional and medical service costs for the elderly, while Medicaid provides similar coverage for the poor; the remainder pay on a sliding scale according to income. On Lok financing is creative. As noted earlier, before joining the program each prospective participant must qualify for nursing home care as determined through an independent assessment by a state representative. Then the government funds On Lok on a fixed per month per capita basis. The level of funding is based on 95 percent of what the government would have had to pay for nursing home care via the Medicare and Medicaid programs. As of 1987, this worked out to a per capita level of about $1,900 per month per participant, which is not a huge difference from what Ontairo Nursing Homes and Homes for the Aged receive for semiprivate accommodation. On Lok uses this money to help keep their participants out of institutions and living in the mainstream of life. The payment allows On Lok great flexibility in program design. They don't have to specifically use their revenue for institutional and physician services, and by and large they don't. In fact, the program is so successful, despite the characteristics of the participants I've described, that at any given time only 6 percent of those participating are in institutions. Contrast that figure with the 10 percent of all Canadians over the age of sixty-five who are in institutions, of which 5 percent are in nursing homes and 1 percent are in acute-care hospitals. They've turned funding on its head. Looking at a comparison of proportional funding 1985–86 between the Ontario Ministry of Health and the On Lok Care program, the latter spent 14 percent on outpatient medical care, while the Ontario Ministry of Health spent 17 percent, which is only a little more. With respect to administration, On Lok does spend a lot more (9 percent) than the Ontario Ministry of Health (1 percent) because they have to deal with private insurers to a great extent. About 0.5 percent of Ontario's funds are spent on research and development, while 7 percent of On Lok funding is used for that purpose. Then look at real differences. Day health services and home care in 1985–86 in Ontario account for 1.7 percent of the budget; in On Lok it accounts for 46 percent. Institutional care for the Ontario Ministry, including physician services within hospitals, absorbed 64 percent of its budget but only 14 percent of On Lok's. I think this program shows that our present funding pryamid can really be turned on its head. Of course, institutional care will always be required, but more and more I believe that services are going to be delivered in noninstitutional settings like On Lok. I think that our system may start moving toward an On Lok-type model, toward a vertically integrated structure, with home and community and institutional services financially linked. Voluntary cooperation is important but a lot of the time it doesn't work that well. To really get things to move smoothly, the different players in the system must be financially linked. This is what I see in the system that we're gradually developing across the country for our health system.

We're moving toward a tri-level health-care system. Ontario has had a Premier's Council on health strategy since 1987, Quebec has been operating with some of the functions of the Premier's Council for several years. New Brunswick, in April (1990) announced the creation of a Premier's Council on Health; Nova Scotia, in March, announced the creation of a Provincial Council on Health that will convene later in 1990. An Ombudsman's office with similar functions to a provincial health council was recommended in the Alberta Premier's Commission, and I think this is a trend that we'll see across the country. There will be some kind of interministerial committee that will deal with an overall strategy for health and will be responsible for setting goals.

On the other hand I can see another trend, which is the regionalization of the day-to-day operation of the health-care system. Quebec developed a regional system in 1970; sometime between 1995 and the year 2000 its fourteen regions will have budgetary responsibility for their respective health-care systems. Ontario is beefing up the power of its district health councils. Alberta's report recommended regional systems, as did the reports in Saskatechewan, Nova Scotia, and New Brunswick. Over the next ten to twenty years we're going to see that happen. The department of health will be left with setting an overall budget for health care, setting minimum standards for their regions, setting a per capita formula for disbursement of funds to the regions, coordinating interregional cooperation, establishing technological assessment and liaison with other provinces and the federal government, as well as licensing and a number of other functions. I think that's the direction in which we're going to be moving; that kind of system will better support the flexibility of funding for long-term care as well, and will allow the trade-offs that are so necessary. In other words, if a region can bring in the proper programs to stop poisoning their seniors with prescription drugs, then that money shouldn't just go back to the provincial government. Instead, it should stay within the region and be used to improve the health of seniors. It should be used to provide better community programs. That opportunity to reallocate is the key, because if you know there's twenty million dollars in your region to be reallocated and if you do something to improve prescribing by your physicians, there's a tremendous incentive to bring in a proper program.

3

Choices: Resource Allocation in the 1990s

Russell Carr

Resource allocation has always been about choices. My argument is that in the 1990s resource allocation is going to be the result of a lot more choice made by a lot more people than it has ever been in the past. If I had been asked to present my views three or four years ago, I would have explained how governments make funding decisions, and how they allocate financial resources across the various sectors of public policy. In the last two or three years, however, I have come to believe that the processes by which public policy gets made are changing dramatically. Critical resources allocated in today's society include more than just financial resources, and these allocations are increasingly made in marketplaces, not in cabinet meetings.

My thesis is that any organization in the 1990s, whether in the public sector, the private sector, the so-called third sector (which includes not-for-profit organizations) will flourish, survive, or fail depending on its ability to allocate three particular resources. The first is financial resources, the traditional focus of resource allocation. The second is human resources; the more labor-intensive an organization is, the greater that challenge will be. The third is the resource of public opinion. What do various publics think will be critical to the survival of organizations of all types in all three sectors in the 1990s? Organizations are going to have to redefine the way they think about planning, management, and policy development in order to ensure that they survive in marketplaces that are increasingly competitive with regard to the allocation of these resources.

ENVIRONMENTAL TRENDS

To begin, I want to scan the environment quickly, specifically to reference six trends that have emerged relevant to the competition for financial, human, and public opinion resources. Some I will wish to review as examples to underscore a general point, while others have particular relevance to the long-term care industry.

The Global Economy

The trend toward a competitive global economy has implications for organizations in the public sector and in the third sector just as much as it does for the private sector. If the business units within our private sector are not competitive and cannot realize income, then income is not available for redistribution to other sectors. With globalization, nationalization is diminishing and developments in all sectors globally will affect us sooner or later, positively or negatively.

The Environmental Movement

The growth of the environmental movement has become a dominant force in recent years. In the next five to ten years it will continue to be of very real significance. The public's concern about issues such as environmental health will continue. Air pollution, water pollution, and recycling will gain profile on the public agenda. Of late, all kinds of business units are scrambing to identify with the public's environmental agenda.

The Animal Rights Movement

A new social movement has emerged around animal rights, and its members are actively lobbying for support. Animal rights organizations are concerned with issues such as the rearing of veal calves and have placed full-page ads in major magazines protesting their treatment. McDonalds Corporation has asked suppliers of chicken products to inform it of the conditions under which chickens are raised, obviously anticipating the need to respond to concerns about the quality of life of these animals. Alert business units do not underestimate the potential impact of public opinion in this area.

The Health and Safety Movement

Right behind the environment movement and the animal rights movement is emerging a health and safety movement. In the workplace, health and safety are going to be major issues of human resource management in the 1990s. In the future when we talk about organizations being competitive in the area of human resources, i.e., their ability to recruit and maintain necessary human resources, an organization's "track record" in health and safety is going to be a major competitive factor. In Alberta, the Premier's Commission on Health Care in their "Rainbow Report" has stated that the health-care industry has a particular responsibility to be a role model in this area.

The Human Rights Movement

Since the 1960s we have become increasingly concerned as a society with human rights. This concern has taken the form of employment equity, legislation, the Charter of Rights,* and/or provincial bills of rights. This growing emphasis on human rights is critical in the human service industry, because it reflects a growing concern with the rights of people to make decisions about their own lives. Issues around independence and empowerment are a fundamental part of the whole rights movement and a major issue in human services in the 1990s.

Changing Demographics

Our population is aging and, as one consequence, its demands for health-care services are likely to increase. However, the availability of human resources to provide that service is likely to decrease. Thus, while the potential marketplace from which labor is purchased is contracting.

TRENDS AND MARKETPLACES

What can we learn from this brief review of these six trends? I think the following lessons emerge.

---

*Refers to those long-term care or nursing home facilities that spell out in their contract the residents' rights and the rights of the facility.

Competitiveness in the Business Marketplace

The first lesson is that competitiveness in the business marketplace will remain intense. Here I am using the term "business" to refer to an organization's field of endeavor, for example, providing long-term care services regardless of whether they are provided by a for-profit or not-for-profit organization. One way in which this competitiveness will be expressed is through pressures to limit the redistribution of financial resources from the private sector to fund such services. It will also be expressed through demands for improved customer service as consumers and their families increasingly expect and demand higher levels of service. It will also be expressed as demand increases for service alternatives that promote empowerment and individualized programming. As universal programs shrink, people will assume more responsibility for their own long-term care through private insurance, employee benefits, and the like. More and more often it will be the case that service providers will satisfy consumers/purchasers rather than funders.

Competitiveness in the Labor Marketplace

The second lesson is that competitiveness in the labor marketplace will increase as traditional labor pools contract with changing demographics. Employers will compete to become "employers of choice." Expectations of employees with regard to quality of work life will increase. Concerns with health and safety issues will be important considerations in determining this quality of work life. So will the nature of employee benefits provided by employers. Benefits, such as day care, will become much more popular in service industries that depend on working mothers as a source of labor. Employers will be competing to recruit and maintain employees who will be with them for a long time—in labor relations, high turnover will replace high cost as the predominant problem. Keeping workers will be less costly than being left without workers.

Competitiveness in the Marketplace of Public Opinion

The third lesson we can learn from the examples of the environmental movement and the animal rights movement is that public opinion in today's world can be mobilized literally overnight. Organizations whose values and practices are thought to be consistent with those of particular interest groups can expect consumer boycotts, demonstrations, and/or pressures on government for intervention. Such government intervention may take the form of regulation and/or reduction in funding support.

A specific point in Alberta is the degree to which long-term care is provided through institutional options, compared to other jurisdictions and in light of growing public support for in-home services.

THE NEED TO REDEFINE MANAGEMENT

My next argument is that, traditionally, we have not defined management in a way that helps us to compete in these three marketplaces. Management theory, as it has traditionally been defined, emerged from disciplines such as industrial engineering, micro-economics, and finance. The art and science of management has thus been defined in technical, quantitative terms, where systems and procedures are really aimed at managing "the human factor" out of any enterprise. Today most organizations still reflect this management style through a primary focus on strategy, structure, systems, and technology, as well as policies and procedures.

This traditional definition of management has often blinded us to the necessity of managing to the realities of human behavior. It is in this context that I reference the insight of Noel Tichy, a professor, author, and consultant in the field of management. In his book *The Transformational Leader,* Tichy argues that organizations successful at transformational change, i.e., responding to the rapidly changing realities of today's world, have enjoyed leaders who managed the political and cultural issues within organizations, not just the technical ones. Political issues within organizations are those dealing with changes or perceived changes in the allocation of commodities such as resources, status, or compensation. Cultural issues are those dealing with the impact of change upon prevailing values and attitudes.

In our consulting practice at William M. Mercer Limited we have found Tichy's insights to be of tremendous value. In most of our assignments we undertake an issues analysis where we examine, not just the technical challenges confronting an organization, but the political and cultural issues as well. This technical/political/cultural (TPC) issue analysis represents substantial "value added" to our clients, who generally lack the social science training we bring to the analysis. The utility of this TPC analysis has demonstrated itself in both specific organizational interventions and more general public policy development. Organizational interventions are those where the challenge of change is focused on changing the behavior of a closed social community, for example, a private corporation. Our work in public policy development on the other hand focuses on changing the behavior of many different social communities or even the general public.

To give an example of the "value added" that comes from TPC analysis, I will reference some of the work we have done in the rehabilitation field. In Alberta we have a Premier's Council on the Status of Persons with Disabilities. We have undertaken work for the council where we have talked with persons with disabilities, advocacy groups, service agencies, and professional groups. One reality emerges from our discussions with these people: driving change in this area is largely a consequence of dealing with the existing value and attitudinal base held by politicians, professionals, and those running service organizations. Each of these groups has very set frameworks in their minds of how they see persons with disabilities. Sometimes, in fact most times, they are not conscious of these frameworks. However, the clients usually are. What is the point of the example? Simply that changes in the delivery of services to persons with disabilities will not primarily be a result of change in policy programs or funding. Rather, it will come from changing the values and attitudes of policy makers, service deliverers, and the general public. Cultural issues, not technical issues, must be the focus for those who would lead change in this area.

To review the argument to this point, successful organizations in the future will be those who can secure customers from an increasingly competitive business marketplace, employees from a shrinking labor marketplace, and public support from an increasingly volatile public opinion marketplace. Fundamental success in all these cases is an ability to understand human behavior and manage in the context of that behavior. Where traditional management theory and practice aimed at managing "the human factor" out of the equation, today's management challenge is to manage it in. The realities of human behavior have to be accommodated by today's organizations as they become increasingly dependent on positive relationships with customers, positive relationships with employees, and positive relationships with the public.

A FOCUS ON HUMAN RESOURCES

Where does this argument now lead us? If the "old management" will not promote competitiveness in these three marketplaces, what management approaches will? Obviously, no simple or single answer can guarantee success within the long-term care industry or any industry. However, success in the future will definitely *not* be experienced by organizations that do not place a high priority on human resources. At the minimum, that priority needs to be expressed in the following ways.

Clarity of Purpose

Today's organizations are generally aware of the value of a purpose or mission statement as a base for planning or management decision making. However, in my experience many organizations do not ensure that the implications of the statement are communicated to the organization's human resources. Unless an organization's human resources understand the behavioral implications of an organization's mission and demonstrate the mission in their behavior, the mission statement alone will have minimal impact.

A Priority of Customer Service

Today's organizations need to ensure that their clarity of purpose reflects a high priority on customer service. They need to ensure that the definition of customer service reflects the customer's perception of service, *not* the organization's. This is a critical point to appreciate in the long-term care field, given the growing emphasis on empowerment and individualized programming.

A True Performance Management System

The behavior implied by the mission statement and demanded by a customer service orientation are so critical to success that they must be reinforced by the performance management system. If the behaviors of staff are deemed fundamental to pursuit of one's mission, and basic to customer service, but are not rewarded by the organization, there is little or no guarantee that these behaviors will be demonstrated by human resources.

Human-Resource Planning

Successful organizations of the future will have in-depth knowledge of the labor pools from which they wish to recruit. They will be aware of the competitive implications of recruiting from this pool and compete accordingly. They will also be aware of the training and development implications of recruiting from this pool and will respond appropriately. They will have become an "employer of choice" within this labor pool and their human-resource programs will reflect the needs of recruits from this pool to become choice employees.

Strategic Benefits Design

Tomorrow's "employees of choice" will provide benefit plans that reflect the needs of the labor pools from which they recruit. For example, those employers who wish to become "employers of choice" for single mothers will increasingly offer child-care services as an employee benefit. Such employers will in turn receive the benefit of improved employee performance. Customer service, for example, is obviously enhanced by employees freed from concerns as to a child's welfare.

In closing, let me review the essentials of my argument. First, when we think of resource allocation in the future we must think of three resources, not one. Second, we must recognize that allocation will increasingly take place in markets, i.e., the business marketplace, the labor marketplace, and the marketplace of public opinion. Third, maintaining competitiveness in all three markets will increasingly be linked to an organization's human-resource practices. These are the realities surrounding resource allocation in the 1990s as I see them.

4

Long-Term Care Policy: A California Dilemma

Linda A. Wray and Fernando M. Torres-Gil

Long-term care means many things to many people. Older people with chronic illnesses and younger people with disabilities perceive it as a health-care issue. Family members who are placing a parent in a nursing home see it is an intensely emotional personal crisis. Providers of long-term care services and products regard it as a burgeoning industry. State and local governments perceive it as a worrisome budget problem. Regardless of one's point of view, long-term care is a public-policy concern that will have major impacts on the short- and long-term fiscal health of national, state, and local governments in the United States.

California faces a slow-motion crisis in responding to the long-term care needs of its citizens. Throughout the 1970s and 1980s, California and the nation grappled with how best to meet the needs of people who were frail, older, and disabled. Federal and state responses to date have been tentative and uneven, due largely to budget deficits and the cost of providing services. Decisive action will become urgent by the turn of the century.

The authors wish to thank Tom Porter, Principal Consultant, California Assembly Committee on Aging and Long-Term Care, for his insights and invaluable comments; and Jeff Hyde, doctoral student, University of Southern California, for his assistance with this chapter's graphics.

The growth in populations of older and disabled persons, and political pressures brought by aging and disability organizations and interest groups, insure that California will be obliged to make important, and often controversial, choices in long-term care policy. California should use the 1990s to plan expansion and reform of its long-term care system before political pressures force hasty and potentially imprudent decisions.

BUILDING BLOCKS OF LONG-TERM CARE

Long-term care is defined as "a set of health, personal care, and social services delivered over a sustained period of time to persons who have lost or never acquired some degree of functional capacity."[1] The ability to perform activities of daily living, such as walking, dressing, and bathing, is central to its definition. Long-term care can also refer to the place in which a service is given (e.g., a nursing home, a board and care facility) or the program that provides the service.[2]

Ideally, long-term care consists of a mix of services—diagnostic, preventive, therapeutic, rehabilitative, supportive, and maintenance—that provide a continuum of care, enabling an individual to stay at home; remain in the community; or, when necessary, find affordable, high-quality institutional care.

The National Picture

The availability of long-term care services in the future will be driven in large part by demographics and public and private sector responses to needs and costs. The aging of the population in the United States, especially the dramatic increase in the numbers of people over eighty-five years of age, is a large part of the demographic imperative. The proportion of people over sixty-five will jump from 13 percent to 20 percent of the population by the year 2030[3]; that population is generally healthier today than previous cohorts of elderly persons. The population eighty-five years of age and over is the fastest growing age group in the country, and it is expected to quadruple between 1980 and 2030.[4] Within that group, health concerns and the need for long-term care are significant.

While most older people with disabilities—approximately 75 percent —are cared for at home,[5] recent trends in family patterns and dependency ratios suggest that fewer caretakers will be available in the home in future years, even though the need for care will be greater. Most older men remain married until they die, and their wives, who have longer life expectancies, generally take care of them when the needs arise. The majority of older women, by contrast, are widowed and live alone, and thus are more likely to require institutional and community-based long-term care. The declining size of the American family, estimated to be less than two children per child-bearing woman in 1990, and the greater numbers of women in the labor force, indicate that there may be fewer adult children to care for older, disabled parents.[6] With today's older people more likely to relocate in their retirement, geographic mobility will also affect the numbers of older people without family and social supports available nearby.

About 21 percent of persons over sixty-five in the United States needed long-term care services in 1988; by the year 2024, this number will increase almost threefold.[7] Barring dramatic medical advances, the need for long-term care among older people will continue to grow.

The California Picture

The growing need for long-term care services in the national population is mirrored in California. In 1985, 11 percent of the state's population were at least sixty-five years old. By 2020 that population will double in size, representing nearly 16 percent of the total population and 65 percent of the long-term care population. Between 1985 and 2020 the population of Californians aged eighty-five and above will grow 145 percent.[8]

In 1985 more than one million Californians, or 39 percent, were estimated to need some type of formal long-term care service. That number is projected to double by 2020.[9] Between 1980 and 2020 the long-term care population is expected to increase at double the rate of growth in the total population. However, factors other than the current rates of morbidity, service use, and mortality, on which these projections are based, may render them tenuous. For example, California's population projections have historically erred on the low side due to underestimates on immigration and mortality.

In addition, the changing racial and ethnic makeup of the California population may also affect the future need for long-term care services. Early in the twenty-first century, California's demographics will shift, and whites will make up less than 50 percent of the population. The groups that have traditionally been considered minorities—blacks, Hispanics, Asians, Pacific Islanders, and Native Americans—are among the most rapidly growing segments of the population. In California, their numbers are projected to increase to at least 40 percent of the elderly population by the year 2020, two and one-half times the 1980 level. As with the total population, the growth of ethnic minorities in the older population will be driven largely by changes in the Hispanic and Asian populations.[10]

Given the current lower usage of health-care services by ethnic minority groups, and their often greater and urgent health-care needs, the extent of their impact on future services is uncertain.

The Nation: A Tentative Response

Currently, there is no national system of publicly funded long-term care services. Instead, there are separate and costly programs that provide a variety of services and benefits. The two largest are Medicare and Medicaid, and each has major gaps and weaknesses.

Medicare, the major source of health insurance for the elderly, primarily covers hospital and physician-based services. While it does reimburse clients for limited home health and nursing home care (when related to prior hospitalization and certified by a doctor), the program was designed to provide acute care rather than longer-term noninstitutional services.

By contrast, Medicaid is the major funding source for nursing home care. In 1987 this program covered 44 percent of total nursing home costs (Medicare and private insurance covered less than 2 percent), while personal out-of-pocket expenditures absorbed the remainder.[11] Unlike Medicare, Medicaid (known as MediCal in California) is a state-administered program that receives matching federal funds. Medicaid is also means-tested, requiring applicants to meet poverty guidelines in order to qualify for services. Despite the program's institutional bias, states may apply for federal waivers to use Medicaid funds for case management and home- and community-based services.[12]

More than eighty other national programs provide long-term care benefits through cash assistance, in-kind transfers, and direct social and health services. Figure 1 demonstrates the tremendous variation in the major national funding sources and services. Each has its own eligibility criteria, oversight agencies, administrative procedures, and requirements.

Despite the existence of these national programs, the major long-term care funding sources for most families are personal expenditures or private long-term care insurance. Family members (usually the women) and friends provide between 75 and 85 percent of direct or indirect long-term care costs. While at least 118 private-sector insurance companies in 1989 offered some form of long-term care insurance in more than 1.5 million policies,[13] private-sector insurance pays less than 3 percent of the total cost of formal long-term care services.[14]

On the national level then, there are a series of large-scale programs, biased toward acute medical care and providing limited supportive services. The United States Congress has proceeded cautiously in expanding community-based chronic care services that may be costly and for

FIGURE 1
FEDERAL FUNDING SOURCES FOR SERVICE NEEDS
OF THE CHRONICALLY IMPAIRED ELDERLY

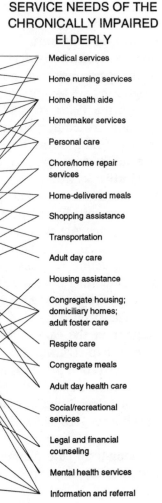

FEDERAL FUNDING SOURCE

Medicaid

Medicare

Social Services

Supplemental Security Income

Administration on Aging

Veterans Administration

Housing and Urban Development

SERVICE NEEDS OF THE CHRONICALLY IMPAIRED ELDERLY

Medical services

Home nursing services

Home health aide

Homemaker services

Personal care

Chore/home repair services

Home-delivered meals

Shopping assistance

Transportation

Adult day care

Housing assistance

Congregate housing; domiciliary homes; adult foster care

Respite care

Congregate meals

Adult day health care

Social/recreational services

Legal and financial counseling

Mental health services

Information and referral

Source: Meyer Katzper, Modeling of Long Term Care   (Dept. of Health & Human Services, 1981), p.16.
In Long Term Care: Who's Responsible?   Critical Debates in an Aging Society, Report No. 2
San Francisco: American Society on Aging, 1988

which the demand is unknown. Recently enacted legislation on nationally funded long-term care coverage has imposed cost-containment measures on Medicare and Medicaid and, where possible, the reduction of coverage and benefits.[15]

California: Restrained Innovation

California has been a pioneer in implementing innovative long-term care services since the early 1970s. Yet the state's attempts to expand and coordinate long-term care funding and services have been restrained by political realities: budget bills require a two-thirds majority for passage in the legislature, and no recent state administration has ever promoted long-term care as a priority issue.

In the 1970s, legislation was enacted to strengthen nursing home inspection procedures; to fund the On Lok Senior Health Services program in San Francisco as an alternative to institutional care*; and to authorize adult day health-care pilot projects funded by MediCal, in-home supportive services and adult day health-care demonstration programs, and waivers from national program requirements to establish the case management Multipurpose Senior Services Program. In the 1980s the Older Californians Act was enacted, comprehensive Independent Living Centers were initiated, Adult Day Health Care centers became permanent programs, and legislation was enacted to improve the quality of nursing home care and allow for second-unit housing or other (what some refer to as "granny flats") shared housing.

The proliferation of national and state funded programs led to an attempt in the early 1980s to reform California's fragmented long-term care system. During that time, the United States Health Care Financing Administration provided a systems development grant to the state to create a plan for a coordinated system of care for impaired Californians. In 1981 the first legislative attempt to develop such a coordinated system was introduced—AB 2860, the Torres-Felando Long-Term Care Reform Act. This bill conferred on the California Department of Aging responsibility for long-term care planning and coordination, and directed the administration to develop a proposal for implementing its provisions.

---

*On Lok began in 1973 as a demonstration program funded by the U.S. Administration on Aging to provide adult day health-care services. This nonpermanent, cost-effective program provides comprehensive long-term care services, including medical care, nursing home placement, social services, in-home care, and housing assistance to its clients in a multilingual and multicultural setting.

However, the incoming administration did not share in the long-term care philosophy of AB 2860, calling its provisions unworkable and prohibitively costly. The refusal of that administration to move forward with the comprehensive statewide coordination called for in AB 2860 led to the introduction by Assemblyman Gerald Felando (R-Torrance) of substitute measure AB 2226. With the support of the administration, AB 2226 passed in 1984, consigning the Department of Aging with "the incremental development of a community-based long-term care system that provides the social and health support necessary to enable frail elderly and functionally impaired adults to remain in their homes."[16]

Today, AB 2226[17] remains the basis for many of the state's long-term care demonstration programs. These programs include Linkages, which establishes regional sites for coordinating services useful in assisting functionally impaired adults to remain in their homes; the "SErvice enrichED" (SEED) community long-term care project, which evaluates different approaches to service integration; and nursing home pre-admission screening programs.

During the 1989–90 legislative session, additional incremental changes in long-term care policy were advanced. Licensure was required for home health agencies that provide skilled nursing services; respiratory therapy in nursing facilities was added to the services covered by MediCal; Medicare Supplemental insurance ("Medigap") consumer protections and standards were implemented; protections were augmented for the elderly in residential care facilities and for consumers buying long-term care insurance; and several demonstration programs, including Linkages, Multipurpose Senior Services Program, and On Lok, were authorized as permanent programs. Additionally, Assemblyman Lloyd Connelly (D-Sacramento) proposed that the state either pass legislation or qualify a ballot initiative establishing a private/public sector program to subsidize the cost of long-term care insurance. Program services, to be financed by a one-half-cent sales tax, included home and alternative care as well as nursing home care. The Connelly initiative was eventually withdrawn due to a lack of support by the state administration and insufficient resources for the signature drive. During the same session, both senate and assembly members introduced several bills relating to the issues of the growing population of medically uninsured, access to affordable long-term care coverage, and health care cost containment.[18]

This two-decade history of long-term care activities in California reveals that the state legislature has attempted, with occasional success, to be innovative in developing services, programs, and coordination mechanisms that use national and state funds more efficiently. The availability of community- and home-based services has moved California closer than the federal government to a balanced continuum of services. However, services have not kept pace with the increasing numbers of older and younger Californians who may need long-term care. Each time the legislature has initiated comprehensive long-term care reforms, it has been checked by uncertain support or recalcitrance on the part of the administration, and held hostage by its two-thirds majority rule on budget bills. Despite the intentions of AB 2226, the state today has a fragmented and uncoordinated array of programs and policies.

California's Fragmented System

The structure and delivery of long-term care services in California reflects the fragmentation of state policy. Figure 2 illustrates the six major agencies under the umbrella of the Health and Welfare Agency that administer the state's thirty-six publicly funded long-term care programs.[19] Those agencies include:

- *California Department of Aging (CDA):* provides supportive services (e.g., nutrition programs, information and referral, an ombudsman, multipurpose senior centers, Meals-On-Wheels) funded primarily by the Older Americans Act; has major responsibility for long-term care policy and planning.

- *Department of Developmental Services (DDS):* administers care, treatment, and training to children and adults with developmental disabilities.

- *Department of Health Services (DHS):* provides medical assistance, including nursing home coverage, to low-income people through the MediCal program.

- *Department of Mental Health (DMH):* provides direct and indirect services to the mentally ill.

- *Department of Rehabilitation (DOR):* assists persons with disabilities through vocational rehabilitation and training programs.

- *Department of Social Services (DSS):* manages income maintenance and social service programs, including in-home support services (IHSS) and food stamps; evaluates disability status for Supplemental Security Income (SSI)/State Supplemental Program (SSP), Medicare and MediCal.

FIGURE 2
State Level Long-Term Care Services: California

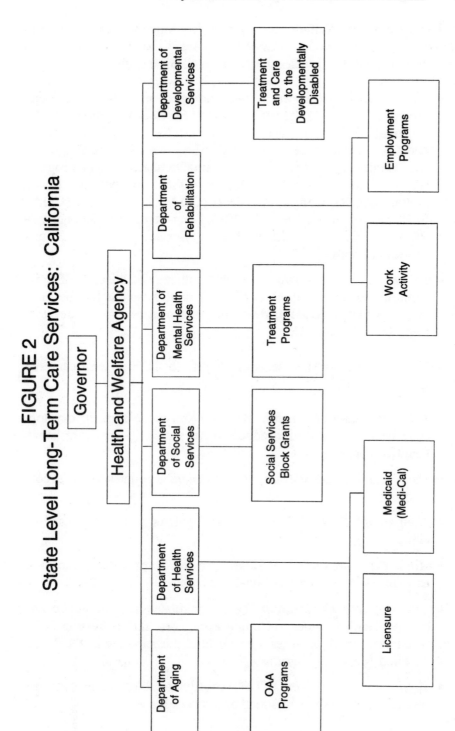

The Health and Welfare Agency classifies long-term care programs as either community-based or institutional care.[20] Examples of long-term care programs (and the agencies that sponsor them) include:

- *Community-based services:* case management (CDA), Linkages program (CDA), Multipurpose Senior Services Programs (CDA), Regional DDS centers, Adult Day Health Care (DSS), Alzheimer's Day Care Resource Centers (CDA), Alzheimer's Disease Diagnostic and Treatment Centers (CDA), Brain Damaged Adults Program (DMH), Adult Protective Services (DSS), Independent Living Centers (DOR), Congregate Meals (CDA), Respite Care (CDA), In-Home Supportive Services (DSS), Long-Term Care Ombudsman Program (CDA), Residential Care Services (DMH), Home-Delivered Meals (CDA).

- *Institutional care programs:* skilled nursing facilities (DHS), institutions for mental diseases (DMH), state hospitals for the mentally disordered (DMH), developmental centers for the developmentally disabled (DDS).

Additional programs and services integral to the long-term care system in California include:[21]

- *Office of Statewide Health Planning and Development:* develops state health policy and conducts surveys of long-term care health facilities' operations and costs.

- *California Medical Assistance Commission:* negotiates MediCal contracts.

- *Community Care Licensing (DSS)* regulates community care facilities.

- *Adult Day Care and Social Day Care (DSS):* provides nonmedical care on a less-than-twenty-four-hour basis.

- *Licensing and Certification (DHS):* regulates licensed public and private health facilities, including acute care, skilled nursing facilities, home health agencies, and facilities participating in the Medicare and MediCal programs.

- *Area Agencies on Aging (CDA):* coordinates Older Americans Act services in thirty-three planning and service areas.

Together these programs accounted for approximately $3 billion of national and state public funds in fiscal year 1987–88. California's share was approximately 40 percent. The five largest programs (MediCal, In-Home Supportive Services, Developmental Centers for the Developmentally Disabled, Regional Department of Developmental Services Centers, Non-MediCal Board and Care) represented 86 percent of the state's total. Approximately 33 percent of the total national and state funding went to the MediCal skilled nursing facility program, compared with 16 percent for the in-home supportive services program.

Despite the substantial public funds expended for this vast array of services, benefits, and oversight activities, California's system has been criticized as a nonsystem of institutionally biased programs.[22] For example, MediCal consumes the largest portion of funds for nursing home care, with the remaining funds divided among thirty-five other programs. The large number of separate agencies involved in designing, regulating, and delivering services has hampered efforts to coordinate that system.

Further, the locus of responsibility for long-term care programs is unbalanced. The Department of Aging, charged with coordinating and overseeing state efforts, consumed just over 5 percent of the long-term care budget in fiscal 1986–87 compared with nearly 35 percent of the Department of Health Services and 27 percent for the Department of Social Services.[23] In addition, relatively few people are served by these programs, despite the state's expenditures on long-term care. For example, the more than $4 million in fiscal year 1986–87 for the Linkages program served only three thousand clients.

POLICY DILEMMAS

The legislative and executive branches in California have responded unevenly to the growing need for long-term care. Despite knowledge of the problems, design, and delivery of long-term care services, the national and state governments and interest groups have approached comprehensive solutions to financing and expanding long-term care with strategies ranging from bold and costly to timid half-steps taken with considerable trepidation.

These responses to the growing needs for long-term care services have been tempered by many policy dilemmas, including: competing social problems, controversies over eligibility and types of service, interest-group politics, financing issues, and questions about service delivery.

Competing Priorities

While the needs of both disabled younger persons and frail older persons are critical, long-term care competes with other priorities that may be more urgent in the short-term. Homelessness, the medically uninsured, AIDS, deteriorating public education, drugs and crime in many communities command immediate attention. The physical infrastructures of highways, bridges, and sewer systems are decaying. Immigrant and refugee groups have pressing needs as well.

To many policy makers, long-term care is a luxury affecting a small number of people rather than a widespread social problem, yet it is likely to evolve into a crisis that affects a large proportion of California's and the nation's citizenry. Policy makers need to understand that greater costs will be incurred by postponing action until the year 2020, when the long-term care population will surge.

Long-term care is subsumed today within the context of national and state health-care coverage. With 37 million Americans (and nearly 20 percent of all Californians) without health insurance, many labor groups, businesses, and consumers are demanding public redress of the health-care crisis. The United States Congress and many state legislatures, including California, are currently weighing bills requiring or encouraging businesses to provide health-care coverage to their employees. However, few of the recent national and state proposals to provide such coverage to the uninsured also cover home- and community-based services. One exception in California is SB 2868, introduced in 1990 by Senator Nicholas Petris (D-Oakland). His comprehensive universal health-care insurance proposal includes long-term care services focused on noninstitutional and case-managed care. Most other California health-care bills limit long-term care coverage to nursing facility care.

Since long-term care issues have traditionally operated on separate advocacy and political tracks from the broader concerns of the uninsured, the absence of coverage today is not surprising. The challenge for long-term care advocates, and in particular the aging network, is twofold: they must broaden their efforts in publicizing long-term care as a problem that affects both elderly and nonelderly; and they must develop alliances with other groups (e.g., the disabled, working uninsured, ethnic minorities, county hospitals, etc.) to insure that health-care solutions incorporate some form of long-term care.

Eligibility and Service Requirements

The development of comprehensive long-term care policy is complicated and politically volatile, especially around issues of eligibility and type of services. For example, most researchers and policy makers agree that an ideal long-term care system permits individuals to choose between home-based, community-based, and medical-based services. Yet, federal policies currently constrain the states' flexibility in promoting social and health services as equal partners.

National studies consistently suggest that the elderly and persons with disabilities prefer to reside in their own homes and communities and use noninstitutional services; however, several factors limit the availability of these services. First, many people do not qualify for In-Home Supportive Services, California's largest publicly funded social service program, and thus must absorb the high costs of private home health and case management services. Second, noninstitutional services may not be less expensive than institutional services; in fact, they may be more costly because they lack the economies of scale of hospitals or nursing homes. Third, the dominant role of physicians indictating the type and duration of treatment often skews services toward medical and hospital-based care.

Determining eligibility for long-term care programs often creates controversy among older and disabled constituencies. Today, most policy analysts and advocates endorse a system that bases eligibility for both programs on limited functional ability (e.g., the inability to perform two or more Activities of Daily Living). While most advocates oppose income- or means-testing for services because it engenders images of a welfare program, most policy makers and budget analysts foresee little choice if costs are to be controlled.

In addition to resolving eligibility and type-of-service issues, policy makers must decide whether the goals of a long-term care system are to promote independence and functional ability or to prevent or stabilize chronic or acute illness.[24] People with disabilities generally prefer the former approach, while older people tend toward the latter. The issue of where to focus expanded services on the individual, the family, or the community also needs resolution. What mix of services and service providers will qualify for participation and reimbursement, and who will maintain control over the disbursement of treatments and services?

A separate and increasingly visible set of issues involves the impact of AIDS patients on long-term care funding for health-care needs. Should policy makers authorize disease-specific health-care programs, or should they expand existing programs to accommodate unforeseen levels of need? During the 101st Congress, legislators considered the allocation of earmarked monies to cities and states and to the Medicaid program for AIDS-related health care. Given current budget constraints, some members were concerned that AIDS care receives a disproportionate share of national health dollars, limiting monies available for all other institutional and noninstitutional care. In addition, some federal policy makers and advocates worried about equity in Medicaid program service delivery in the event that special coverage were permitted for people who are both poor and AIDS-infected.[25]

All of these issues represent difficult policy decisions involving different constituencies, each with a stake in expanding and reshaping a long-term care service system. An ideal scenario for those needing services, of course, would be a universal entitlement program, qualifying all persons regardless of income, age, or disability, for noninstitutional case-managed, and institutional care, and all providers and programs for reimbursement. That scenario, financed in part through payroll taxes and copayments, is currently embedded in California Senator Petris's SB 2868, introduced in 1990. Because of its sweeping changes and costs, the future of that bill in the state legislature is uncertain.* However, anything less than a universal program will require hard choices and trade-offs.

Interest-Group Politics

Who will influence the development of long-term care policy in California and in the nation? Who will address technical and administrative issues in service delivery? Decisions on need, priorities, and types of services require confronting the relative political influence of various constituencies.

Senior Citizens: Older people and the organizations that represent them are often powerful forces on national, state, and local levels. Their power was evidenced most recently by the rapid formation of a grassroots movement that forced Congress to repeal the Medicare Catastrophic Coverage Act of 1988, which would have expanded Medicare and Medicaid benefits.[26] That event demonstrated a political truism: while senior citizens may not be able to promote legislative funding or expansion, they can halt the implementation of unpopular legislation and proposals.[27]

Similarly, in California, policy makers take seriously the concerns of senior citizens, who register and vote at higher rates than do other segments of the voting-age public. Key groups advocating on behalf of older Californians include the umbrella Senior Coalition, the California Rural

---

*Senate Bill 2868 died without final action at the end of the 1989-1990 legislative session. Reintroduced in 1991 as SB 36, the bill will be heard in January 1992 in the Senate Revenue and Taxation Committee.

Legal Assistance Foundation—Senior Program, the Congress of California Seniors, the American Association of Retired Persons, and the Gray Panthers. In addition, the California Commission on Aging affords senior citizens access to the governor. The California Senior Legislature also focuses on influencing the state legislature.

Persons with Disabilities: Persons with disabilities in California have an equal interest in the politics of long-term care. The population at least sixteen years of age who have disabilities is estimated at nearly 11 percent of the total state population; about 75 percent of these people can be classified as severely disabled.[28] Both overall disabling conditions and those that are severe are more prevalent among women and minorities than among men and nonminorities.

Although the communities of the elderly and the disabled share preferences for independent living, home-delivered services, and comprehensive health-care coverage, the specific interests of the two have not always coincided. The community of those with disabilities also has a system of programs separate from those of the elderly community. Because these programs focus on rehabilitation rather than on receiving care, people with disabilities, and the advocacy groups representing them, may prefer that long-term care services for the elderly and those for the disabled remain separate. Earlier proposals to merge program funding within the state departments of aging and rehabilitation caused consternation among both senior citizen and disabled groups.[29] If developing a cost-effective system requires merging long-term care programs, the preferences and system investments of the two communities will remain major issues in the debates. Clearly, in order to minimize group struggles, both communities must be involved in each phase of policy formulation.

Other Players: Interest by other groups in the politics of long-term care has increased in recent years. The personal nature of long-term care, the issues associated with financing services, and the diverse community of advocacy and professional groups affected by this care ensure that other players will continue to be concerned with long-term care policy.

While many national and state minority organizations consider long-term care a priority issue, sources of public funding have been limited for programs designed to provide such care to meet the needs of ethnic minorities. Given the growing numbers of minority elderly, their greater likelihood of facing chronic illness, and their preference for home and community services, long-term care is certain to become more critical to them in the future.

Decision Makers: Long-term care policy will not be decided by interest groups, academicians, legislative staffs, elected officials, or civil servants alone, even though many are delegated with varying levels of authority for policy formulation and implementation.

At the national level, the agency charged with Medicare and Medicaid oversight and regulations is the Health Care Financing Administration (HCFA), whose director reports to the secretary of health and human services. Legislative jurisdiction over long-term care policy matters is shared among committees in the Senate and the House of Representatives, as illustrated by figure 3; California currently has several members of Congress on these committees.

At the state level, there is no single agency analogous to HCFA, in which regulatory, financing, and oversight actions are lodged. Instead, the Office of Statewide Health Planning and Development is charged with developing state health policies and surveying long-term care facilities. The Department of Aging is the lead agency for coordinating long-term care services, which are limited primarily to services, demonstration projects, and waivers consistent with the Older Americans Act. The Department of Health oversees nursing homes funded by MediCal, and the Department of Social Services administers the large In-Home Supportive Services Program.

Historically, the executive branch has provided little leadership on aging or long-term care service issues. Although Governor George Deukmejian (1982–1990) supported some initiatives aimed at coordinating long-term care programs, his office did not advance the issues in the long-term care debates. And while staffs of gubernatorial campaigns were briefed on long-term care issues by assembly staff in 1990, no candidates from either party elevated the issues to priority status.

In recent years, while the legislature attempted to pursue long-term care legislation, it has been successful in maintaining bipartisan support only on small, incremental changes. Few comprehensive bills have been enacted due to the lack of support by the executive branch and the two-thirds approval rule on budget matters. Aside from the initiatives introduced by Chairperson Lloyd Connelly (D-Sacramento), of the Assembly Committee on Aging and Long-Term Care, few members of committees with jurisdiction over such matters (e.g., the Senate Subcommittee on Aging and Long-Term Care, the Senate and Assembly Committees on Health, and the Committees on Appropriations) were visible in the long-term care policy debates on comprehensive care services until 1990. During that year, Assemblyman John Vasconcellos (D-San Jose) of the Committee on Aging and Long-Term Care and Chairperson Bruce Bronzan (D-Fresno) of the Assembly Committee on Health introduced legislation related to long-term care.

Given the historically disjointed attention to long-term care in California government, who, then, is responding today to the growing pressures associated with providing and financing services? Because of budget

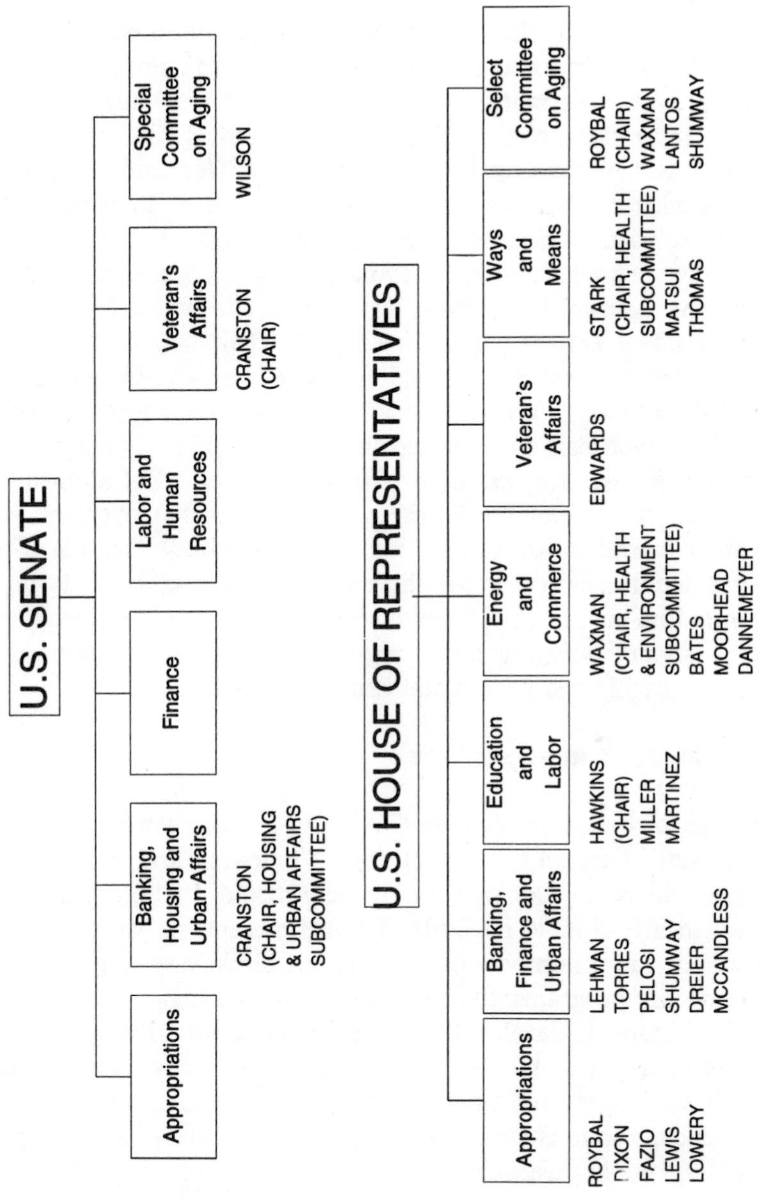

FIGURE 3
REPRESENTATION OF CALIFORNIA CONGRESSIONAL DELEGATION ON COMMITTEES WITH JURISDICTION OVER LONG-TERM CARE ISSUES

U.S. SENATE

Appropriations	Banking, Housing and Urban Affairs	Finance	Labor and Human Resources	Veteran's Affairs	Special Committee on Aging
	CRANSTON (CHAIR, HOUSING & URBAN AFFAIRS SUBCOMMITTEE)			CRANSTON (CHAIR)	WILSON

U.S. HOUSE OF REPRESENTATIVES

Appropriations	Banking, Finance and Urban Affairs	Education and Labor	Energy and Commerce	Veteran's Affairs	Ways and Means	Select Committee on Aging
ROYBAL	LEHMAN	HAWKINS	WAXMAN	EDWARDS	STARK	ROYBAL
NIXON	TORRES	(CHAIR)	(CHAIR, HEALTH		(CHAIR, HEALTH	(CHAIR)
FAZIO	PELOSI	MILLER	& ENVIRONMENT		SUBCOMMITTEE)	WAXMAN
LEWIS	SHUMWAY	MARTINEZ	SUBCOMMITTEE)		MATSUI	LANTOS
LOWERY	DREIER		BATES		THOMAS	SHUMWAY
	MCCANDLESS		MOORHEAD			
			DANNEMEYER			

constraints, the national government has moved cautiously. Congress, the Department of Health and Human Services, and affected interest groups continue to engage in extended debate about solutions to the long-term care dilemma.

Reacting to the slow progress at the national level, several states, including California, run consumer education and counseling programs to provide information on public and private long-term care programs and insurance policies. Eight states, including California, are pressuring the U.S. Congress for waivers to combine Medicaid coverage with private insurance against the costs of long-term care. In general, these public-private partnerships would encourage the growth of the private insurance market according to state standards, and encourage consumers to buy private insurance. For both insurer and consumer, Medicaid would serve as a safety net—if consumers exhaust their benefits, they would qualify for Medicaid without "spending down" to poverty; thus, insurers know Medicaid would ultimately bear the costs of their more expensive cases.

Waiver legislation passed the U.S. Senate in 1989, but is still pending in the House. Representative Henry Waxman (D-California), the powerful chairperson of the House subcommittee that oversees Medicaid, and other members are said to be concerned about the role of Medicaid as a potential safety net for the middle class, taking Medicaid funds away from low-income people, and the possible costs of the programs.[30]

Again, hovering over long-term care service definitions and politics is the prickly and paramount issue of financing.

Paying for Long-Term Care

Costs of long-term care in California are projected to continue spiraling upward. Assuming constant 1986–87 dollars and a base model, projection, the state Department of Health and Welfare estimates that costs will nearly double by 2020. If those projections were revised to account for the large numbers of persons not already served by the state's long-term care programs, the costs would be even higher.[31]

Figure 4, developed by the Institute for Health and Aging at the University of California at San Francisco, presents alternate public and private options for financing the projected long-term care costs. Public financing options include incremental expansions of public programs, voluntary public insurance, and mandatory public insurance. Private funding options focus on private long-term care insurance.

The national government has inclined toward a combination of public and private financing: augmenting Medicare and social services to expand respite and nursing home days and home care under the Older Americans

FIGURE 4
PUBLIC POLICY OPTIONS FOR LONG-TERM CARE IN CALIFORNIA

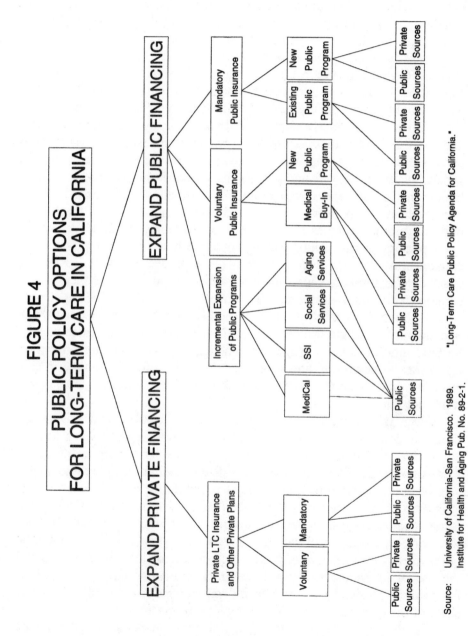

Source: University of California-San Francisco. 1989.
           Institute for Health and Aging Pub. No. 89-2-1.

"Long-Term Care Public Policy Agenda for California."

Act; using Medicare and MediCal waivers for case management and community-based services; and proposing Medicaid buy-in programs, in which individuals purchase private insurance with assurance of qualifying for Medicaid when private coverage expires. Potential funding sources include payroll taxes, general revenues, value-added taxes, selected excise taxes (e.g., on alcohol and tobacco purchases), income tax surcharges, and liens on estates. The option advanced most often (included in the Pepper/Roybal home care bill that was defeated in 1988) would lift the cap on the Social Security payroll tax wage base (currently set at $51,000), which would provide an estimated $6 billion per year for health care.

With a larger elderly population that is, on average, more affluent and healthier today than in the past, private long-term care insurance is perceived as an important option. However, private insurance is not yet widely available, and many policies have other shortcomings, such as limitations in care and coverage and high monthly premiums. In addition, even under the most favorable economic circumstances, the Brookings Institution estimates that in the year 2020 only 26 to 45 percent of older persons in the United States would be able to afford private coverage against the catastrophic costs of an extended disability.[32] Recently enacted legislation in California was aimed at moderating these shortcomings. These bills—introduced by Senators Henry Mello (D-Santa Cruz), Alan Robbins (D-Van Nuys), and Assembly Member Lloyd Connelly (D-Sacramento)—include prohibitions against clauses requiring three days of hospitalization prior to payment of benefits, policy cancellations based on age or health condition, and consumer protections for the long-term care insurance market similar to those enacted for the Medicare supplemental insurance market.

Given the strengths and weaknesses of both public and private options, cooperation between the public and the private sectors is a feasible alternative, one that is currently being pursued by a number of states. For example, public funds might subsidize the voluntary purchase of private insurance premiums. States might mandate the expansion of private long-term care policies or the addition of long-term care services in existing medical insurance policies, or provide incentives to purchase private long-term care insurance that meets state standards.[33] The national government's examination of private long-term care insurance policies and the use of individual retirement accounts and home equity conversions for medical purposes, delegate to individuals and their families a larger share of the responsibility for financing long-term care needs.

Clearly, these developments suggest that financing long-term care services may be costly in the short-run, but what will be the costs of doing nothing? Proposed financing options will be directly affected by the perception of long-term care as a priority social need and by the political actions of interest groups, decision makers, and the public.

Recent state and national opinion polls indicate that strong public support exists for public funding of long-term care. A recent Gallup California Health Care poll indicated that 65 percent of Californians believe government is spending too little for the care of senior citizens; and 73 percent would pay additional taxes to support the health care of those in need.[34] Whether these findings translate into political support for increased taxes for long-term care services remains an open question.

Service Delivery

An additional issue concerns the structure of long-term care service delivery at the local level. Expansion of existing services will directly affect the city, county, and state agencies that provide the services.

The complex and fragmented laws, regulations, and financing sources administered by multiple agencies of the federal and state governments result in equally complex, fragmented, and often inaccessible services in the community. For example, in general, county departments of health oversee nursing homes, while county departments of social services have jurisdiction over the In-Home Social Services programs, and city and county area agencies on aging coordinate other long-term care services. In addition, private, for-profit home-care programs proliferate in many more affluent areas. Only recently did the state impose operations standards for board and care facilities that provide housing for individuals who might otherwise be institutionalized.

This array of unconnected services heightens the critical importance of effective case management; information and referral services; and written understandings among state, county, and city agencies. In response to that need, some localities (e.g., Los Angeles County) have promoted cooperation across the city, county, and private sectors through long-term care task forces.

Major expansions of long-term care services will impel fundamental reforms in service delivery and a major restructuring of existing programs. Like reforms in financing, those in service delivery are likely to be difficult. For instance, legislation in the early 1980s proposing the coordination of services through a state long-term care corporation or through area agencies on aging generated significant and intense interagency disputes.

Other issues that will affect local service delivery include the availability and specialized training of health and long-term care personnel. By the year 2000, approximately 50 percent more physicians, nurses, occupational and physical therapists, geriatric social workers, case managers, gerontologists, and mental-health workers will be needed than are available today in order to fully staff all forms of health and long-term care services to the elderly.[35] While geriatricians are in short supply today, the recent granting of board certification and the presence of selected geriatric medical programs (e.g., at the University of California-San Francisco, the University of California-Los Angeles, the University of Southern California, and Stanford University) may ameliorate that situation in the future.

Service Needs of Ethnic Minorities

Finally, several present and potential characteristics of minority elderly populations have major implications for long-term care policy in California. First, because of lower income levels, the capacity of today's elderly minorities to pay for health and long-term care is limited. For example, Mexican-Americans, the predominant Hispanic group in California, have the highest proportion of medically uninsured persons in the United States (30 percent, compared with 9 percent of white non-Hispanics).[36] Without improvements in present income patterns, significant portions of California's minority population will confront serious problems in assisting their elderly parents and financing their own long-term care needs. Second, minority elderly are more likely to need long-term care because of tendencies toward chronic illnesses that may start at earlier ages than in the white population.

Strong family and informal support networks are common among ethnic minorities,[37] and minority elderly are less likely to reside in long-term care facilities than are nonminority elderly. However, it is uncertain whether these patterns will continue in the future, given the trends toward assimilation, upward mobility, and geographic dispersion.

POLITICS OF LONG-TERM CARE

Current long-term care policy dilemmas point out the inherently political nature of such care and the difficult choices that lie ahead. Both the national and state governments will wrestle with the complexities of the financing and delivery of needed services in the next few decades.

The repeal of the Medicare Catastrophic Coverage Act of 1988 appears to have stymied the movement toward development of a comprehensive national long-term care system in the near future. In fact, one of the key factors leading to the grassroots opposition to the legislation was its exclusion of long-term care insurance coverage. After the repeal, national policy makers shifted their attention to other policy issues, citing the federal deficit, the need to contain escalating health-care costs, and concern for the uninsured as obstacles to serious consideration of costly expansions of Medicare and Medicaid long-term care. At the state level, budget deficits have encouraged efforts to contain costs by reducing services.

Nonetheless, long-term care issues remain on the public agenda at both national and state levels. Many of the health-care bills introduced in the 101st Congress provide for additional funding for home- and community-based care.[38] The Elder Care Long-Term Care Assistance Act (HR 3140), introduced in 1989 by Representative Henry Waxman (D-California), proposes in-home long-term care services and nursing facility care under Medicare. Senator Edward Kennedy (D-Massachusetts) introduced a Lifecare bill (S 2163) in 1990 that would provide home care to elderly persons, disabled children, and Medicare-eligible disabled adults under age sixty-five. Both bills would finance the programs by eliminating the Medicare payroll tax wage cap. The Medicare Benefit Improvements Act (HR 3880), introduced in 1990 by Representative Fortney Stark (D-California), would reauthorize the expanded mammography, home health-care screening, respite and hospice benefits lost in the repeal of the Medicare Catastrophic Coverage Act. These benefits would be fully financed by a modest increase in the Medicare Part B premiums.

In California, the passage of Proposition 111 in June 1990, loosening previously imposed state spending constraints, will allow California more flexibility in spending for health and aging services. However, that flexibility will result in intense competition among advocates for long-term care and those seeking coverage for other health and social needs.

Short-Run Prognosis

The prospects for short-run resolutions are limited. The executive and legislative branches on both national and state levels are preoccupied with the politically popular health-care issues of the medically uninsured and national health insurance, which are generally considered separate from long-term care. The Congress is likely to consider, but unlikely to adopt, proposals to improve the quality and financing of nursing home care and to develop publicly funded community- and home-based services. Policy makers will continue to debate whether a universal national health-care system can afford to include long-term care services. Thus, long-term care likely will remain a secondary issue in the foreseeable future.

The repeal of the Medicare Catastrophic Coverage Act of 1988 illustrates the impasse. To some the repeal fueled a growing backlash against older persons and the share of the federal budget devoted to programs for them, along with a shifting allegiance toward children and the poor. To others, it was a temporary setback that will be forgotten by the 1992 congressional and presidential elections, during which the electoral power of older people will recast long-term care into an important political issue. More likely, unless a dramatic political event elevates long-term care to primary status, we will see continued incremental expansion of publicly funded long-term care.

Long-Run Prognosis

The long-run outlook is more promising for a comprehensive long-term care service system. Demographic pressures, increasing numbers of people with disabling conditions (particularly among women and ethnic minority populations), the aging of the baby boomers, the escalating electoral clout of those groups, increased geographic mobility, and changes in living arrangements will command the attention of governments and propel the development of a comprehensive long-term care service system.

Within ten years, we can expect public funding of coverage for a continuum of home- and community-based services for younger and older people with at least two or three functional disabilities. Such a system will include means-testing and cost-sharing provisions for low- and middle-income groups, and cost-containment mechanisms. Private medical insurance, governed by strict state standards, will be expanded to include a range of long-term care services; public funds will subsidize the purchase of such policies on a sliding income scale. In addition, tax incentives will encourage private-sector businesses to provide expanded dependent care benefits for caretaking of both children and disabled parents.

Strategies

Because of California's special demographic circumstances, the state may not have the luxury of waiting for federal action on long-term care. It must proceed soon with a structural strategy as well as incremental reforms, despite the inherently politicized nature of long-term care. The new governor's office and the legislature should work closely with the powerful California congressional delegation to shape joint federal-state strategies, ensuring that federal proposals meet California's needs.

The framework for a coordinated system was authorized in Assembly Bill 2860, and recent legislative activity on health insurance and long-term care suggests an atmosphere of greater awareness, discussion, and urgency. The new administration is in an enviable position to court an increasingly large electorate—the diverse population of baby boomers and their families—by taking a leadership role on the long-term care issue.

Interest groups and others concerned with health and long-term care should continue to negotiate the basic features of a statewide long-term care system. Task forces, universities, and advocacy groups should convene long-term care "summits" and come to agreement on recommendations for policy changes. Some of the issues to be considered have been proposed by the National Council on Aging: shared responsibility between the national and state governments; universal eligibility, signifying a multigenerational approach to long-term care service; a social insurance approach to financing; and inclusion of housing, social services, and rehabilitation as integral services.

The long-term care service system must build upon and coordinate existing services and set minimum standards for them. Area agencies on aging are logical candidates for coordinating the services in the community, while the state Department on Aging has greater latitude and administrative authority to plan and oversee state-level programs. Culturally sensitive programs and successful projects—such as On Lok, the Multipurpose Senior Services Program projects and Linkages—should be continued and expanded. With political pressures building in support of long-term care, California universities must produce the personnel needed to staff long-term care programs.

In addition, California must educate the public about the implications of increased life expectancies and the very real possibility that most people will need long-term care at some point in their lives. In order to moderate needs and costs, the state must also encourage consumer education on financing long-term care and preventive health-care practices; gerontology instruction in high schools and colleges; and congregate-care facilities and other alternative living arrangements.

California policy makers and advocates must use the 1990s as a decade of opportunity to prepare for the next century's long-term care needs. Electoral support for expanding the long-term care service system will emerge in the near future. In California, that support may manifest itself in a long-term care services initiative by 1992. The nation and the state will be forced to confront the diverse needs of expanding older and disabled populations, the political interests of baby boomers and their elected officials, and the complex dilemmas associated with coordinating and financing a continuum of long-term care services.

NOTES

1. Rosalie Kane and Robert Kane, *Long-Term Care: Principles, Programs and Policies* (New York: Springer, 1987).

2. Ibid.

3. U.S. Senate, *Aging America: Trends and Projections,* 1987-1988 edition (Washington, D.C.: Department of Health and Human Services.)

4. Ibid.

5. See Kane and Kane, *Long-Term Care: Principles, Programs and Policies.*

6. U.S. Bureau of the Census, Current Population Reports, Series P-25, No. 1018, *Projections of the Population of the United States by Age, Sex and Race: 1988 to 2080,* by Gregory Spencer (Washington, D.C.: U.S. Government Printing Office).

7. American Society on Aging, "Long-Term Care: Who's Responsible?" in *Critical Debates in an Aging Society,* Report No. 2. (San Francisco: American Society on Aging, 1988).

8. Health and Welfare Agency, *A Study of California's Publicly Funded Long-Term Care Programs* (Sacramento, Calif.: Health and Welfare Agency, 1988).

9. Institute for Health and Aging, *Long-Term Care Public Policy Agenda for California,* Pub. No. 89-W-1 (San Francisco: University of California, 1989).

10. Fernando Torres-Gil and Jeffrey C. Hyde, "The Impact of Minorities on Long-Term Care Policy in California," in Liebig and Lammers (eds.), *California Policy Choices for Long-Term Care* (Los Angeles: University of Southern California, 1990).

11. Congressional Research Service, *CRS Issue Brief: Long-Term Care for the Elderly,* Pub. No. IB88098 (Washington, D.C.: Congressional Research Service, Library of Congress, 1990).

12. Legislation directing the application of waivers for that purpose was introduced in 1990 by California Assemblyman Burt Margolin (D-Los Angeles).

13. Torres-Gil and Hyde, "The Impact of Minorities on Long-Term Care Policy in California."

14. University of California-San Francisco, *Long-Term Care Public Policy Agenda for California.*

15. For example, a prospective payment system established in 1983 and a relative value scale added in 1990 were designed to control expenditures in the Medicare program by setting predetermined reimbursement rates for hospital and physician services according to geographic area and types of services.

16. California Department of Aging, *Request for Proposals for Linkage Sites in Accordance with AB 2226* (Sacramento, Calif.: Department of Aging, 1985).

17. Welfare and Institutions Code, Chapter 1637, 1984 Statutes, Division 8.5, Section 9390.

18. The major health insurance bills were introduced by California Assembly Speaker Willie Brown (D-San Francisco), Assembly Members William Baker (R-Walnut Creek), Bruce Bronzan (D-Fresno), Dan Hauser (D-Eureka), Burt Margolin (D-Los Angeles), and Senators Ken Maddy (R-Fresno) and Nicholas Petris (D-Oakland).

19. Health and Welfare Agency, *A Study of California's Publicly Funded Long-Term Care Programs.*

20. Ibid.

21. Ibid.

22. Assembly Office of Research, "The Graying of California: The Third Shock Wave," in *California 2000: A People in Transition* (Sacramento, Calif.: Assembly Office of Research, 1986).

23. Health and Welfare Agency, *A Study of California's Publicly Funded Long-Term Care Programs.*

24. Tom Porter, Principal Consultant, California Assembly Committee on Aging and Long-Term Care.

25. Julie Kosterlitz, "Is Support for AIDS Slipping?" *National Journal* (June 2, 1990): 1351.

26. Fernando Torres-Gil, "The Politics of Catastrophic and Long-Term Care Coverage," *Journal of Aging and Social Policy* (1): 61–86.

27. Robert Binstock, Martin A. Levin, and Richard Weatherley, "Political Dilemmas of Social Intervention," in Binstock and Shanas (eds.), *The Handbook of Aging and the Social Sciences* (New York: Von Nostrand Reinhold, 1985). See also William Browne and Laura K. Olsen, *Aging and Public Policy* (Westport, Conn.: Greenwood Press, 1983).

28. J. M. Shanks and H. E. Freeman, *Executive Summary for the California Disability Survey* (Sacramento, Calif.: Department of Rehabilitation, 1980).

29. Fernando Torres-Gil and Jon Pynoos, "Long-Term Care Policy and Interest Group Struggles," *The Gerontologist* 26, no. 5: 488–495.

30. Julie Rovner, "No Help from Congress on a Near-Term Solution for Long-Term Care," *Governing* (June 1990).

31. Ibid.

32. Alice Rivlin and Joshua Wiener, "Who Should Pay for Long-Term Care for the Elderly?" *The Brookings Review* 6, no. 3: 3–9.

33. Alaska, Ohio, and South Carolina currently offer long-term care insurance to their state employees and retirees, with the enrollees paying

the full premium costs. Unlike other long-term care proposals described earlier, federal waivers are not required in order to provide coverage to their own state employees.

34. Institute for Health and Aging, *Long-Term Care Public Policy Agenda for California,* Research Brief No. 7 (San Francisco: University of California-San Francisco, 1989).

35. Employment Development Department, *California Projections of Employment by Industry and Occupation: 1987-2000* (Sacramento, Calif.: California Employment Development Department, 1990).

36. F. M. Trevino and A. J. Moss, "Health Insurance Coverage and Physician Visits among Hispanic and Non-Hispanic People," in *Health, United States, 1983,* National Center for Health Statistics, DHHS Pub. No. (PHS) 84-1232, Public Health Service (Washington, D.C.: U.S. Government Printing Office, 1983).

37. R. J. Taylor, "Aging and Supportive Relationships among Black Americans," in Jackson (ed.) *The Black Elderly: Research on Physical and Psychosocial Health* (New York: Springer, 1988). See also M. Sotomayor and A. Curiel (eds.) *Hispanic Elderly: A Cultural Signature* (Edinburg, Tex.: Pan American University Press, 1988); Louise Kamikawa, "Expanding Perceptions of Aging: The Pacific Asian Elderly," *Generations* 6, no. 3 (1982): 26-27; Carmela G. Lacayo, *A National Study to Assess the Service Needs of the Hispanic Elderly: Final Report* (Los Angeles, Asociacion Nacional Por Personas Mayores, 1980).

38. Torres-Gil and Hyde, "The Impact of Minorities on Long-Term Care Policy in California."

5

Empowerment and Aging

Mark Novak

INTRODUCTION

I want to begin with a game that I call "Social Issues Bingo." Write down the five most serious problems that you think older people face today. Now compare the issues you have listed with findings from a poll by the George Harris organization in the United States. This poll asked a random sample of younger and older people to comment on older people's problems.

Compare the proportion of younger people and older people who considered an item a very serious problem. In every case a greater proportion of younger people thought an item was a very serious problem. Also note that more older people thought these were serious problems for other older people than actually reported these problems themselves. Both younger and older people, it seems, have a negative view of aging, and younger people have a more negative view than older people. The Harris poll findings suggest that one of the worst problems older people face today is the attitudes of other people toward aging.

The popular culture often supports this negative view of aging. Advertising, television, and jokes often give a negative slant to aging. Birthday cards, for instance, make direct comments about how people feel about aging. Often these cards make jokes about failing health, de-

TABLE 1

HARRIS POLL (1981) RESULTS

"Very Serious Problem" (%)

	Felt Personally	Expected by 18-64	Expected by 65+
Poor Health	21	47	40
Lonely	13	65	45
Not Enough Money to Live On	17	68	50
Poor Housing	5	43	30
Fear of Crime	25	74	58

cline in sexual vigor, and loss of beauty. One card expressed this negative feeling openly. It said, "Roses are red, violets are blue, thank goodness I'm not older than you."

A health-care equipment representative in my area recently gave me a list of comments about aging titled "You Know You're Getting Old." The list includes the following items. You know you're getting old when: You sink your teeth into a steak and they stay there; you look forward to a dull evening; you turn out the lights for economic rather than romantic reasons; a fortune teller offers to read your face. These items get a chuckle out of most people. But a closer look shows that they play on our prejudiced feelings about aging. These comments focus on the supposed loss of control and power that comes with age. This includes the loss of control of our own bodies (a decrease in sexual ability, gusto in eating and drinking, and attractiveness). The use of humor disguises the effects of these comments. They make older people seem foolish and less capable than the young. They distance younger people from the older person by making the older person different. And they provide some justification for taking control and power from older people as they age.

Empowerment occurs when an activity, social structure, environmental design, or social relationship enhances people's abilities to define their own interests, decide their own course of action, and act to control their own destinies. I believe this power stands as a basic human right. But I know that a person in a powerful position—a teacher, a health-care worker, an administrator—can inhibit other people's power to act. This happens in horrible places like concentration camps, prisons, and mental hospitals. But it can also happen in hospitals, personal care homes, and elder residences. A health-care professional can rob someone else of power just as effectively as an unjust political regime. But in the health-care system it's done in the name of care, kindness, and concern. An aging society challenges us to find ways to care for older people and at the same time leave them with the power to act and make choices for themselves.

Here I will present:

(1) some of the facts about the aging of the older population in Canada;

(2) some of the issues and challenges that will face long-term care professionals in the future;

(3) some of the ways we can empower the people we serve.

Many caregivers work in institutional settings, but I will also discuss empowerment and long-term care in noninstitutional settings. Some of the trends and issues in an aging society argue against focusing on institutions when we think about long-term care. Empowerment should include giving the older persons the choice to stay out of institutions.

THE SECOND DEMOGRAPHIC BOOM—THE SENIOR BOOM

Sometimes the future rushes in on us in some ways we least expect. Demographers noticed the post-war baby boom only after it happened. And this population bulge has changed North American society. Likewise, demographers have just begun to notice a second population trend that will influence society—the decline in mortality rates at the oldest ages. Leroy Stone, Senior Statistician at Statistics Canada, calls this "the second most consequential development (after the baby boom) in the recent demographic history of developed countries."[1]

Figure 1 shows the increase in life expectancy for men and women eighty years of age from 1926 to 1971.

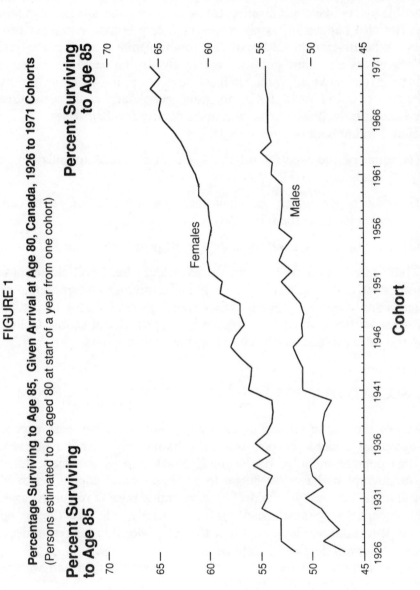

FIGURE 1

Percentage Surviving to Age 85, Given Arrival at Age 80, Canada, 1926 to 1971 Cohorts

(Persons estimated to be aged 80 at start of a year from one cohort)

Source: Leroy O. Stone and Susan Fletcher.   The Seniors Boom. Statistics Canada. Catalogue Number 89-515. Chart 3.3. 1986.
Adapted with the permission of the Minister of Supply and Services Canada. 1991.

Women have gained more in life expectancy than men over this time. But both sexes now show an increase in the percent of eighty-year-olds who survive to age eighty-five.

This decline in mortality will lead to more older people. In the 1980s the seventy-five-plus groups showed an annual increase in size of at least 3.5 percent per year (the largest increase in the older population), and more people were reaching the very-old age group (eighty-five-plus). Stone and Fletcher (1986) report that the group eighty-five and older, for instance, will grow proportionally faster than any other age group in Canadian society between now and the year 2011 (4 percent per year during 1991–2001; 3 percent per year from 2001–2011). Older age groups will also increase in size. A rising proportion of older people today and in the future will live into their nineties and hundreds.

What will this mean for long-term care and for the empowerment of older people? Demographic change tells only part of the story of seniors' future need for empowerment within the long-term care system. We need to match these demographic facts to what we know about older people's changing abilities as they age.

HEALTH AND ABILITIES WITH AGE

Health

The 1985 Canadian General Social Survey (GSS), published in 1987, asked a random sample of all community-dwelling Canadians aged fifteen and over about their health. The survey found a dramatic increase in self-reported health problems as we age (see table 2, page 72).[2]

Health and Welfare Canada and Statistics Canada (1981) reports that almost 90 percent of people aged sixty-five or older suffer from a chronic illness. About 50 percent of people aged sixty-five or older suffer from arthritis or rheumatism, and an estimated 9 percent have diabetes.[3] Note that a greater proportion of people aged sixty-five or older, compared to the general population, reports having each of these chronic illnesses—sometimes by as much as three or four to one.

TABLE 2

CANADIAN GENERAL SOCIAL SURVEY (1985)

Reported Health Problems (%)

	Males		Females	
	All Ages	*65+*	*All Ages*	*65+*
Hypertension	15	33	17	43
Heart Trouble	7	28	7	24
Diabetes	2	9	3	9
Respiratory Problems	10	26	12	23
Arthritis/ Rheumatism	17	46	26	63

Source: Statistics Canada, *Health and Social Report, 1985* (Cat. No. 11–612), Ottawa: Minister of Supply and Services Canada, 1987, Table 51. Adapted with permission of the Minister of Supply and Services, Canada, 1991.

Functional Ability

The GSS also reports that functional disability increases with age.

TABLE 3

GENERAL SOCIAL SURVEY, (1985)

Degree of Activity Limitation (%)

	Males		Females	
	All Ages	*65+*	*All Ages*	*65+*
Moderate	3	13	5	18
Major	1	6*	2	12

* = high sampling variance, use with caution.
   Source: Statistics Canada, *Health and Social Report, 1985* (Cat. No. 11–612), Ottawa: Minister of Supply and Services Canada, 1987, Table 40. Adapted with permission of the Minister of Supply and Services, Canada, 1991.

Thirteen percent of men and 18 percent of women aged sixty-five or older report moderate activity limitation. Twelve percent of women in this age group report major activity limitation. The use of seventy-five or eighty years as a cut-off would produce even greater differences between the oldest age groups and the general population.

Now we can bring together these facts on demographics, illness, and disability. Figure 2 (see page 74) presents another look at the impact of longer life on aging. It shows the rate of decline of three groups of Canadians over time. The more current the group, the slower the rate of decline. The most recent group's curve describes a population that survives almost intact until old age and then dies off relatively quickly. Demographers refer to this pattern as the rectangularization of the life curve. Figure 2 shows this life curve and a hypothetical curve of a group's decrease in functional ability.

Figure 2 allows us to raise an important question. Will the curve of disability follow the curve of life expectancy as life expectancy increases? In other words, will future groups show delays in the onset of disability that corresponds to delays in mortality?

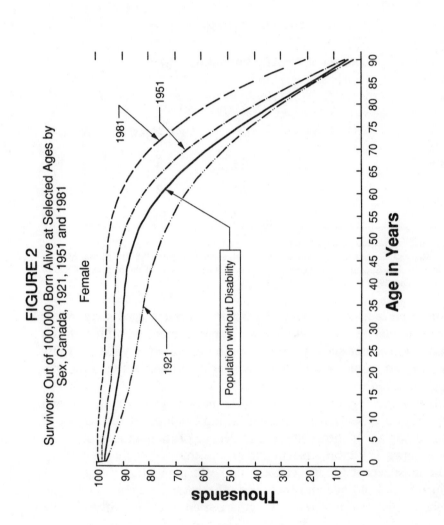

FIGURE 2

Survivors Out of 100,000 Born Alive at Selected Ages by
Sex, Canada, 1921, 1951 and 1981

Female

1981

1951

1921

Population without Disability

Age in Years

Thousands

Source: Dhruva Nagnur. Longevity and Historical Life Tables. Statistics Canada, Catalogue number 89-506, p.74, Chart C4
Adapted with the permission of the Minister of Supply and Services Canada, 1991.

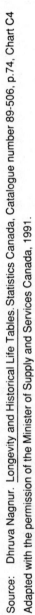

Fries says that longer life expectancy has come about through decrease in such chronic illnesses as smallpox, whooping cough, and diphtheria.[4] In the future, he says, decreased rates of chronic illness in old age—lung cancer, stroke, and heart disease, will lead to longer life. He also says that this holds out the chance for a postponement of illness until late old age ("the compression of morbidity").[5] It will lead to a longer and healthier life.

But some writers challenge this optimistic view of the future. Simmons-Tropea and Osborn say that "the major causes of morbidity are *not* necessarily related to the major causes of mortality."[6] Manton says that chronic degenerative (but not necessarily fatal) conditions cause the most disability.[7] These conditions include the most common illnesses reported by older people: diabetes, respiratory problems, and arthritis/rheumatism. People live with these last few diseases for many years. This could lead to larger numbers of people than ever before living with severe functional impairment.

No clear answer to this controversy exists. Canadian data do not support Fries's prediction. These data show no decrease in the proportion of people in poor health as the population has increased in life expectancy. Instead, the data suggest that people will live longer with chronic diseases. In Canada, from 1951 to 1978, for instance, life expectancy increased 4.5 years for men and 7.5 years for women. For this same period, disabled years increased by 2.9 years. This means that Canadians made only small gains in "disability free years."[8] They conclude that "these data strongly suggest that the years gained in life expectancy will be largely spent suffering long-term activity limitation. Less than 30 percent of the increased years of life expectancy from 1951 to 1978 can be expected to be free from limitation."[9]

Disability and declining mobility threaten the quality of life in old age. People with disabilities will more likely have low perceived health, more physician consultations, more hospitalizations, and need more housework done for them.[10] As the population ages, this problem will affect more and more people, and it will increase the demand on health and social services. It will put more and more older people under the care of health-care professionals and institutions.

How can leaders in the field of long-term care respond to this challenge? How can we empower the large number of older people who face decreases in health and activity?

THREE STRATEGIES FOR EMPOWERMENT IN AN AGING SOCIETY

I propose three strategies to empower older people now and in the future:

1. environmental adaptation;

2. health promotion;

3. education for life enrichment.

Each of these strategies leads to empowerment of the individual. Each encourages, demands, or allows the older person to control his or her destiny.

1. Environmental Adaptation

Canada has one of the highest institutionalization rates in the world for older people. On any one day in Canada in 1981, for example, almost 6 percent of men and 9 percent of women aged sixty-five and over lived in health-care institutions (nursing homes and hospitals).[11] Some provinces have even higher rates.

As the population ages, and the proportion of people with disabilities increases, the numbers and proportion of older people who spend some time in a Canadian institution could increase. This would be an unfortunate development because a number of studies show that institutionalization can lead to decreased well-being and even death for older residents.[12] Other studies show that institutionalization leads to high health-care costs.[13]

Government leaders, doctors, nursing home staff, and the elderly themselves agree that we should keep older people out of institutions when we can. A case study of one woman will show some of the ways to help older people stay at home.

Mrs. Chalmers, seventy-seven, lives in a one-bedroom apartment in Winnipeg. Her husband died seven years ago and she has lived alone in their apartment since then. She lives on the third floor of a forty-year-old apartment building. It has no lobby, no social services, no amenity space, and no elevator. She finds it harder each year to walk the steps to her apartment. She now goes down only once a day to check her mail. In the winter she stays in unless her daughter drives her to a shopping mall. Her daughter lives two hours away by car and comes to visit about once every three weeks.

Mrs. Chalmers sees her doctor about every six weeks. Between visits she uses no health-care services. She takes medication for her high blood pressure and arthritis. She watches her diet because of a slight rise in her blood sugar. Three years ago she came down with jaundice, and she had phlebitis in her legs. Since then Mrs. Chalmers has had no serious illnesses. She does all of her own housework, cooking, and personal care. A cleaning woman comes in once a month to do a thorough cleaning.

Mrs. Chalmers has many friends. She talks to them on the phone nearly every day. As she ages, though, she sees her friends less and less. Some of them are also widows. They never learned to drive, and in winter none of them get out very much. Mrs. Chalmers also talks to her son and his family every two weeks. They live on the East Coast and visit her (or she visits them) about once a year. She plays the role of kin-keeper for her family and this gives her a sense of purpose.

Mrs. Chalmers generally stays in good spirits, though she sometimes worries about her health and finances. She also worries about simple things like how to get food. She finds it hard to walk to the store and even harder to carry her groceries up to her apartment. Her superintendent helps sometimes, but she doesn't like to impose on his good will. She wishes she could do the things she used to do. Mrs. Chalmers has pretty well given up going to the store on her own. She says she's getting too old to do that now.

Typical of many older people her age, Mrs. Chalmers is widowed, she lives alone, and she has at least one health problem. She also has two of the most common health problems reported by Canadian women over the age of sixty-five—hypertension and arthritis/rheumatism. Mrs. Chalmers has begun to face some risks in her present setting. (1) She risks psychological decline because her informal support network has shrunk (due to loss of her spouse, loss of mobility, and her friends' similar losses). (2) She risks dietary deficiency because she can't buy food when she needs it and because she has no one with whom she can share meals. (3) She risks atrophy of her strength because she goes out less and less.

Mrs. Chalmers can no longer function optimally in her environment. Her social support network has changed, her health has changed, and she has begun to feel fatalistic about her life as she ages. ("I have to depend on everybody to do for me now," she says.)

What can or should be done to help Mrs. Chalmers? What can we do that will increase her ability to make choices and act on her own? What general principles about empowerment can we apply to her or to seniors like her?

Lawton and Nahemow designed a diagram that presents some principles for empowerment.[14] It offers a model of what they call Person-

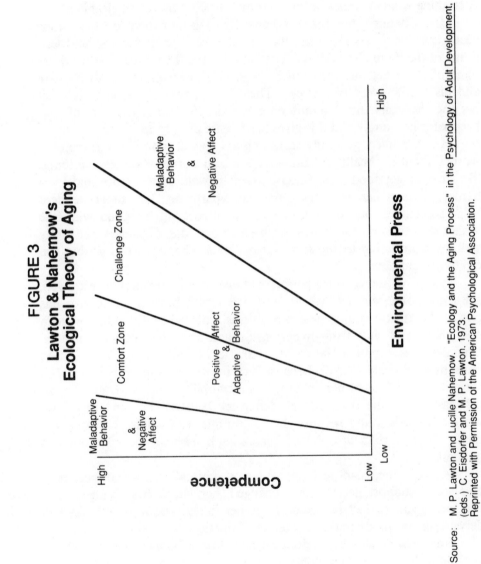

FIGURE 3
Lawton & Nahemow's
Ecological Theory of Aging

Source: M. P. Lawton and Lucille Nahemow. "Ecology and the Aging Process" in the Psychology of Adult Development.
           (eds.) C. Eisdorfer and M. P. Lawton. 1973.
           Reprinted with Permission of the American Psychological Association.

Environment fit. It helps us to see how we can address the changing needs of people as they age and increase their decision-making power.

Figure 3 shows two dimensions of person-environment fit: individual capability (competence) and the demands of the environment (environmental press). Note that the higher the competence the greater the range of press, and that low competence makes a person more susceptible to changes in press. This means that a small environmental change (e.g., a homemaker) could lead to an improvement in how well a person can manage at home. Note that an optimal environment includes a balance of challenge and abilities, and that too little press is as bad as too much. This model teaches an important lesson. Environmental support must change to meet changing competence. Aging is a dynamic process that requires assessment, modification, adaptation, and reassessment.

Figure 3 suggests certain approaches that empower older people. *First,* beware of too little press. Be aware of isolating the older person in a cocoon-like environment. *Second,* note that we can increase competence as well as decrease press. An increase in competence pays off in more adaptability over a broad range of demands. *Third,* adaptation can take more than one path. Older people should play a role in designing and choosing their own options.

What has happened to Mrs. Chalmers since I first saw her in August, 1988? She moved the following September to a senior's residence. She still cooks and does most of the cleaning herself, but has a woman come in once a month to do heavy cleaning. She now attends movies on Saturdays, sits in the residence lobby each afternoon, and goes to dinners and parties in the building. A van takes her shopping twice a week, and someone helps carry her bundles to her door. She has made new friends who visit her. This spring she plans to go with her friends to a senior center at the end of their street. Today she says she lives, "a different life, a better life." Mrs. Chalmers has maintained her lifestyle and her sense of independence. She has even developed some new interests and new relationships.

In *Successful Aging* I described Lions Place, an eighteen-story apartment building for seniors in Winnipeg. This building includes amenities and programs that make it a model for seniors' housing.[15] On the ground floor, for instance,

> potted ferns and small trees are set alongside lounge-chairs in front of floor-to-ceiling windows. . . . Behind this lounge stretches over 5,000 square feet of space with card-tables, soft chairs for reading or relaxing, and more plants. At the back of the lounge stands a two-story humdi-

fied greenhouse where tenants can take classes in gardening and where they can care for their own plants.[16]

The east wing of the building houses a beauty salon, a craft shop, a convenience store, an extension branch of the public library, and space for a small geriatric clinic with examination rooms.[17] The second floor has an exercise room, a whirlpool, a sauna, and changing rooms. It also has a kitchen and a dining room that seats 150 people. Each floor has a tub room that can accommodate a person in a wheelchair. The Lions Club built these amenities for present and future use.

Most of the tenants today manage their own personal hygiene and cook for themselves in their apartments. But, as tenants age and lose some physical abilities, they will be able to use the public dining room and get assistance with bathing.

Lions Place provides supports, but it also works to increase tenants' competence. Tenants profit from a full-time recreation staff, which helped set up a residents' council. This council plans activities for the tenants and attempts to make Lions Place a challenging and socially active environment. Through good planning, design, and management, Lions Place helps older people enjoy life and stay in their own apartments as long as possible.

Housing should help older people to function well and maintain their lifestyle. It should help them meet their basic needs. But empowerment goes beyond basic needs. It also includes opportunities for growth, personal development, and self-actualization.

2. Health Promotion

"The majority of the aged remain functionally well until an advanced age."[18] Studies of seniors in both Calgary[19] and Saskatchewan,[20] for example, found that 60 percent of seniors report good or excellent health. Health promotion and postponement of chronic illness would lead to a decrease in the years of disability. Some of the newest approaches to keeping people well also help them to get more out of life.

In 1981, Health and Welfare Canada set up a Health Promotion Directorate to "inform and motivate people to adopt and maintain healthy lifestyles."[21] A new program designed by the directorate for seniors, called *Discover Choices,* shows what a health-promotion program offers.

This program aims to "encourage older adults to make informed choices about their health by increasing their knowledge of the lifestyle, social, and environmental factors that affect health and quality of life."[22] The government, after talking with agencies and aging specialists, targeted this program to Manitoba and Saskatchewan seniors aged fifty-five to seventy-four, with low incomes ($10,000 for single people, $18,000 for families), and low education (grade 10 or less).

The program includes a series of twelve half-hour television programs on current health and lifestyle issues, twenty-four articles on health topics written mostly by seniors, media promotion materials, and community development projects. The program encourages existing seniors' groups to act as resource and referral centers as well as consultants to the Health Promotion Directorate. The program and an evaluation study of its effect began in September, 1988.

Canada has only begun to value the health promotion model of health care. But health promotion seems to have caught on among seniors. Statistics show that more older people exercise today than in the past. Able-bodied seniors (sixty-five years of age and over) show a greater increase in exercise participation from 1976 to 1981 than any other age group. Also, 30 to 40 percent of older men and women reported eating fewer fatty and fried foods in the past year than in previous years.[23] Healthier lifestyles and habits will increase older people's competence and decrease the incidence of chronic illness. This should help keep the elderly out of institutions.

3. Education for Life Enrichment

Later life means more than physical decline, adaptation, and survival. Gerontologists now generally agree that people can learn, develop their personalities, and enjoy new experiences at every age. We empower people when we give them the ability to learn, grow, and develop regardless of their phsyical condition. This poses challenges for education in the future.

One group has already begun to take up this challenge. Creative Retirement Manitoba (CRM), a seniors' learning center in Winnipeg, runs dozens of courses for seniors. CRM has a board of directors composed entirely of seniors and the elderly teach most of the classes. The programming includes: reflexology, massage, reminiscence workshops, dream analysis, a distinguished professors series, a harmonic band, calligraphy, and Tai Chi team. Creative Retirement will face a new crisis this fall due to population aging. It will not have enough Tai Chi teachers to meet the demand of students who want this program.

Creative Retirement has also begun to look to the future. Its own population of students has aged in the past ten years. Many students cannot get out in the winter. *Homebound Learning Program* has therefore been started to meet the needs of people who cannot come to classes. A facilitator assesses a person's learning needs in their home. Then an instructor (usually a senior volunteer) comes to the home to offer the classes. Classes include classical literature, conversational French, and micro-computer use. This program and others, including teleconference courses, televised education in senior residences, and classes in senior residences will all develop in the future.

SUMMARY

The three approaches described above—increased environmental support, healthier lifestyles, and more chances for self-development—can all em-power older people and meet the future challenges of an aging Canadian population. These approaches fit with a new view of later life. We now know that people can grow, develop, and learn at every age. And geron-tologists recognize that growth and development happen most often in a supportive social environment. The latest trends in housing, health promotion, and education show how people can live to a *good age* in an aging society.

NOTES

1. L. O. Stone and S. Fletcher, *The Seniors Book* (Ottawa: Minister of Supply and Services, Statistics Canada Cat. No. 89–515E, 1986), Section 3.1.

2. *General Social Survey Analysis Series, Health and Social Support* (Ottawa: Minister of Supply and Services, Statistics Canada Cat. No. 11–612, 1987) No. 1.

3. Ibid.

4. James F. Fries, "Medical Perspectives upon Successful Aging," in Paul S. Baltes and Margaret M. Baltes *Successful Aging: Perspectives from the Behavioral Sciences* (Cambridge: Cambridge University Press, 1990).

5. James F. Fries, "The Elimination of Premature Disease," in Ken Dychtwald and Judy MacLean (eds.) *Wellness and Health Promotion for the Elderly* (Rockville, Md.: Aspen, 1986).

6. Daryl Simmons-Tropea and Richard Osborn, "Disease, Survival and Death: The Health Status of Canada's Elderly," in Victor W. Marshall (ed.) *Aging in Canada,* 2d ed. (Toronto: Fitzhenry and Whiteside, 1987).

7. Kenneth G. Manton, "Post and Future Expectancy Increase at Later Ages: Their Implications for the Linkage of Chronic Morbidity, Disability, and Mortality," *Journal of Gerontology* 41 (1986): 672–68.

8. Simmons-Tropea and Osborn, "Disease, Survival and Death."

9. Ibid., p. 419.

10. *General Social Survey Analysis Series, Health and Social Support* (1987).

11. Statistics Canada, 1984.

12. See Neena L. Chappell and Margaret Penning, "The Trend away from Institutionalization: Human or Economic Efficiency?" *Research on Aging,* 1 (1979): 361–87; Gloria Gutnam and C. P. Herbert, "Mortality Rates among Relocated Extended Care Patients," *Journal of Gerontology* 31 (1976): 352–57; Gloria Gutman, C. Jackson, A. J. Start, and B. Mc-Cashin, "Mortality Rates Five Years after Admission to a Long-Term Care Program," *Canadian Journal on Aging* 5 (1986): 9–17; M. J. MacLean and R. J. Bonar, "The Ethnic Elderly in a Dominant Culture Long-Term Care Facility," *Canadian Ethnic Studies* 15 (1983): 51–59.

13. *The Health of Canadians (The Canada Health Survey).* (Ottawa, Minister of Supply and Services, 1981), Health and Welfare Canada and Statistics Canada Cat. No. 82–538; Frank T. Denton and B. G. Spencer, "Population Aging and Future Health Care Costs in Canada," *Canadian Public Policy* 9 (1983): 155–63.

14. M. Powell Lawton and Lucille Nahemow, "Ecology and the Aging Process," in Carl Eisdorfer and M. Powell Lawton (eds.) *The Psychology of Adult Development and Aging* (Washington, D.C.: American Psychological Association, 1973).

15. Mark Novak, *Successful Aging: The Myths, Realities and Future of Aging in Canada* (Markham, Ontario: Penguin, 1985).

16. Ibid., p. 122.

17. Ibid.

18. "Canadian Governmental Report on Aging," *Health and Welfare Canada.* (Ottawa: Minister of Supply and Services), p. 43.

19. *A Profile on the Elderly in Calgary: A Demographic Profile and Needs Assessment* (Calgary: City of Calgary, Research and Planning Unit, Family and Community Support Services Division, Social Services Department, 1983).

20. *Choosing a Special Care Home in Saskatechewan* (Regina: Senior Citizens' Provincial Council, 1983).

20. Signy Hansen and G. Ledoux, "Developing a Health Promotion Resource for Older Adults." Paper presented at the Meeting of the International Association of Gerontology, New York, 1985.

22. Health and Welfare Canada. *Discover Choices* (pamphlet.) (Ottawa: Minister of Supply and Services, 1988).

23. Stone aned Fletcher, *The Seniors Boom.*

REFERENCES

Manton, Kenneth G. (1986). "Past and Future Life Expectancy Increases at Later Ages: Their Implications for the Linkage of Chronic Morbidity, Disability, and Mortality." *Journal of Gerontology* 41:672–81.

Fries, James F. (1990). "Medical Perspectives upon Successful Aging." In *Successful Aging: Perspectives from the Behavioral Sciences,* eds. Paul B. Baltes and Margaret M. Baltes. Cambridge: Cambridge University Press.

———. (1986). "The Elimination of Premature Disease." In *Wellness and Health Promotion for the Elderly* (ed.) Ken Dychtwald and Judy MacLean. Rockville, Maryland: Aspen.

Schneider, E. L., and J. A. Brody (1983). "Aging, Natural Death and the Compression of Morbidity: Another View." *New England Journal of Medicine* 309:854–56.

Simmons-Torpea, Daryl, and Richard Osborn (1987). "Disease, Survival and Death: The Health Status of Canada's Elderly." In *Aging in Canada, 2nd ed.* (ed.) Victor W. Marshall. Toronto: Fitzhenry and Whiteside.

Statistics Canada (1987). *Health and Social Support, 1985. General Social Survey Analysis Series.* Cat. no. 11–612, No. 1. Ottawa: Minister of Supply and Services.

Lawton, M. Powell, and Lucille Nahemow, (1973). "Ecology and the Aging Process." In *The Psychology of Adult Development and Aging* (ed.) Carl Eisdorfer and M. Powell Lawton. Washington, D.C.: American Psychological Association.

6

Directions for Long-Term Care

Joy Calkin

My focus is on the issue of responsiveness to and recognition of humans in need of help over the long term, and the consumer in the context of organizational decision making. I will share with you where I believe we need to move in the 1990s, and why I believe we need to move there. Part of my thinking comes from my experience as a commissioner on the Premier's Commission on Future Health Care for Alberta, and the opportunity to work with six other special people who dedicated half or more of their seven days a week to the work of the commission. We were supported by a staff and an external group who contributed to our growth and development.

We talked to many people in Alberta at town hall meetings and we heard from several hundred groups concerning their preferences for the future. We began to understand that the consumers were well in advance of providers of care. They were also advanced in their expectations of and hopes for the policy makers in the Province. Indeed, they raised questions and moved further than the commission thought was possible. Some influence on my thinking came from the commissioners meetings with other committees that were mandated to look at long-term care, rehabilitative care, mental illness, and other parts of what falls under the general umbrella of long-term care.

As I look at our health-care system in North America and within

Canada, it is clear that in the last two decades, we have focused on matters of effectiveness and efficiency. To some extent, we have examined quality of life for workers in these organizations. In a more limited way we've paid attention to matters of long-term care public-health policy, but in large measure our writing and our concerns have centered on the matters of effectiveness and efficiency. Some of our problems arise from this emphasis. I do not mean to imply that it is unimportant to pay attention to the patient classification system, or to look at budgets. But I am saying that as we work with residents or with community-based care, much that we do—the tasks we perform, the ways we think—arise from a concern with being more effective in meeting organizational goals and being more efficient in the delivery of services. Florence Nightingale provided a sense of direction when she said we must put an individual in the best place for nature to act upon him.

My focus is on the issue of responsiveness to and recognition of human beings in need of help over the long term, or the consumer in the context of organizational decision making. I'm going to begin with the organization because I think it's out of our concept of the organization —what we think it is and how we think about it—that we make decisions on behalf of human beings who need help.

The present system of long-term care has developed primarily from decisions made by informal organizations—voluntary, publicly funded, and for-profit—about what is meant by long-term care. We need to redefine what *is* long-term care and how systems are to be developed to meet long-term care needs. This does not necessarily mean that we currently use the recognition of and responsiveness to human needs as the controlling decision or direction for long-term care. Sometimes as we try to balance organizational goals, the goals of those who live and work in organizations, and the goals of the consumers of our organizations, decisions conflict. The issue for us is how to develop ways to reduce conflict.

In the study of organizations, we have examined theory and practice to help us better understand those who provide long-term care. We considered a long-term care organization to be a place in which residents or patients or consumers are, according to one theory, "input" to the system. In that *systems view* they are converted into some kind of "output," that is, we have an input of a nonambulatory person and an output of an ambulatory person. What troubles us is what happens during that "throughput." Much writing has focused on the systems view, particularly relating to our support services.

We also viewed long-term care organizations as goal oriented in what is called a *rational systems model*, where people live in an environment from which various resources, including clients or residents, are obtained and in which efficiency must be realized. Measurements must be made and made efficiently. Coordination of providers must be done so as to reduce conflict, and good management is essential to make it all work.

We viewed long-term care organizations according to what's called the natural approach or, more commonly, the *human relations* school. Here the intent is to create an organization in which the aspirations or hopes of the individual members of the community who live and work together are as important as the goals of the board or larger overall administrative group. We studied ways of creating and shaping organizations so that the worker would be recognized. We attended conferences and discussed such issues as participatory decision making, getting your staff "on board and on side," rewarding and sanctioning behavior, and evaluating strategies that helped people become involved and invested in the organization. It was clear that human goals were as important as the measure of workload or hierarchical lines of authority.

Whether one thinks in a *systems model* or in a goals-oriented *rational model* or in a *human relations model* is, I think, less and less important as a central issue or goal. It is important to have a clear sense of a preferred future and the direction for long-term care that flows from a sense of vision. Without a sense of vision and direction, we will not do well in our future.

My argument, then, is a very simple one. When providers and funders are the focus of our thinking and of our activities, we focus on issues such as empowerment, which implies that we must give the power to decide *back* to the consumer. It suggests that as providers or as funders *we* have the power to give back. Many people convince us that power to make decisions was not ours to give, although it was possible for providers and funders to take it away. To deal with long-term care needs, consumers must have the power to influence organizational decision making. To make the necessary changes in the direction for long-term care, the power to make and influence decisions must be put into the hands of consumers. The question for us as providers and funders is "How do we make that happen?"

In our research, which developed the three-volume *Rainbow Report,* we interviewed people with disabling conditions that required long-term care, people in mental health programs, and the Calgary Association for Independent Living (CAIL). In CAIL a group who had needs for long-term care, which providers had not satisfactorily met, developed a pilot program for direct funding. An advocate, who was not a health-care provider, helped the client identify needs and understand community resources well enough so that the client could gain access to those resources. Clearly there was a need for an approach that fosters self-reliance so that a quadraplegic, for example, can exercise the controls necessary in achieving and maintaining autonomy and dignity. Finally, the *Rainbow Report* recommended that in the Province of Alberta the concept of direct personalized payment for persons with special long-term care needs be implemented in community-based programs so as to reduce restrictions to self-defined needs for care while encouraging self-reliance and dignity. Funding would be directly under the patient's control rather than being filtered through a government payment structure. The reasons in back of these recommendations recognized two ways of providing a sense of self-control and dignity:

1. Through knowledge. If the person knows how to care for himself or herself and knows how the system works and how to get care, the ability to exert influence and make decisions is enhanced.

2. Through money. It is clear that people of wealth and substance have power to influence their own health care. Poverty and lack of education are the two factors that have the most negative influence on the health of citizens. A family with a chronically ill child, without the information necessary to make decisions, and without the financial resources to enforce their decisions is seriously disenfranchised.

For those who need assistance with decisions and in finding support and caring, I suggest that CAIL has developed an idea that works—an idea that in some senses hurts my nursing soul, because I think I am the one who ought to advocate for the patients. However, social workers have informed me that they really are the ones who should advocate for the residents. Recently, the chaplains convinced me that they really were the ones who should advocate for the patients. The person at the admissions desk at the Foothills Hospital convinced me that she really was the one who advocated for the patients. It turns out that hardly anyone *really* advocates for the patient. What we do is advocate for our own particular view of human needs for the patients and residents.

How, then, do we shift control of decisions to consumers, with support from "all of us" through our taxes, and from "some of us" through insurance companies? That decision forms a direction for the '90s. It is my view that the most challenging issue in this decade will be the tension between those of us (providers and funders) who really believe we know what residents and consumers need and the consumers who need to be in control and to have a sense of direction over their own life state and their own dignity. Discussion of consumer control has continued throughout my career. I graduated thirty years ago, and from the time that I was a first-year student I heard about how we need to be supportive of patients and how they need to be in control. But at what point do we acknowledge that power differentials occur in our system and that they occur basically because people who need care lack control of the funds or they lack knowledge about how to use those funds and how to allocate them? If I were to challenge consumers, I would urge that through political and other means that we have at hand, we should continue to urge our society to move in the direction of placing decisions in our hands. (I am willing to admit that at the outset I always know better than my patients, and since most are between four and twelve years of age it's not hard to make that assumption. However, I have learned that at least half of the time I'm incorrect as those young children begin to direct and control their own care. I hear them suggest to the pediatrician how they really ought to be managed, and they are often correct.)

If our society is to be responsive and to recognize human needs adequately, then our movement in specific directions must take place in the context of what long-term care means to patients, to doctors, and to caregivers. One hundred years ago, we had three kinds of providers: ward/housekeeper, physicians, and nurses. We now have almost three hundred occupations in the health-care field. We have done a remarkable job of specializing and subdividing our work. But in my childhood, the "nursing home" was in our home. The notions of long-term care, "long-termness of care," and long-term care institutions were more recent concepts and more recent endeavors, except in the care of the mentally ill. We have developed institutions that focus on a range of services from residential living to rehabilitative services. Currently the context has been broadened to identify more clearly community-based care as a firm and necessary component of long-term care. We now see a range of services from community-based care to the intensive care unit, and then in between we have various levels of community-based care and residential, nursing home, or auxiliary services.

Providers and funding agencies control who we are or what we've become. Our future direction must be one of greater individual control. But control of what? How do we design a system for individuals who experience tremendous differences in their needs? How do we create a system that seriously addresses those differences?

How do I help Mrs. Jones find a better alternative to her catheter? How do I make sure that the staff knows how she is to be looked after? We've had written care plans, taped reports, and video communications. Then we put together interdisciplinary teams: we sat down and looked at the long-term care needs of a schizophrenic who is going to live with us for a long time or an individual who is quadriplegic or an Inuit (Eskimo) who has milliary tuberculosis, and we plan the care activities for these people. In some instances we included the person, the resident, or the family in developing plans for care. Somehow, we don't adapt quickly enough or well enough for those with long-term care needs. The resident may have a need or be ready to have that need met, and there's a rigid response that's planned a week or a day in advance.

Somehow providers, consumers, funders, policy makers and all relevant parties must knit the elements of need together in a way that creates a garment that fits each person who is in need of long-term care. Each of us has very different needs, and I think we need to reassess completely the design of our system, for it continues to be too rigid for people and for their changing needs. Part of what has happened is that we have become increasingly invested in our organizational views of community-based care, residential care, and long-term care. Rather than focusing on the person who, for example, may go through a period of acute illness then want to return to long-term care in the community, we may think a nursing home facility would be better. Somehow we have failed to be responsive enough to individual differences.

The question becomes one of determining how to shift the control of decisions to those most affected—to consumers, residents, patients, and their families. First, I would shift the funding. I think it's the most important thing we can do as a matter of public policy. I would urge insurance companies to consider greater consumer control. I would leave the control of payment and other decisions more in the hands of those who require our services and get advice or support for them beyond that of traditional providers. I'm not trying to create another provider in an advocate; I'm simply acknowledging that my view as a provider/administrator may be antithetical to designing a system that is responsive to people. We need to teach, from the time people are in grade school, how the health system does and does not work. If there's anything we learned during the Alberta Commission, it was that people entered our system with virtually no ability to discern what services are available or required.

Now we turn to the notion of direction for the long-term care system. If knowledge and funding is shifted to consumers, will we make it easier for people to convince providers or funders how their care ought to be directed? In the experience we have to date, in the few pilot tests that have occurred where people have more control over the direction of their care and over their funds, they seem to do better in terms of their own quality of life. This is different from when one goes into an intensive care unit; it's different from when one goes to an emergency care setting and is scared to death because of a broken arm, or because one's child has been very badly injured. In these settings we give up much of our control. We're not sure. We can't make decisions. Our minds are not functioning. But that's not true in long-term care. Many of the people for whom we work are perfectly able to make their decisions, and for people who aren't, we're able to find a way to help them make necessary decisions (via their family or their minister or a power of attorney). Will this drive providers and funders to distraction? Did the Alberta Commission really suggest that we give all these people who don't know up from down about the health-care system, the right to spend their own money when they might go out and hire chiropractors? Worse yet, they might hire a Shaman to treat dermatological problems. It is true that some *might* make really bad decisions, but at least they are their own decisions. Historically, providers have made some really poor decisions in health care. (For example, we drove the Obstetrician Samuel Weiss out of his mind because he insisted that when physicians examined women who had died of childbirth infections, they should wash their hands before they went back to the clean part of the hospital [as we think of it now] to deliver women who were having babies. He concluded this from the observation that women delivered by nurse midwives rarely died of childbirth fever because the nurse midwives didn't do pathology examinations on dead bodies that were infected. Germ theory was developed some years later.) As I say, we have made serious mistakes, and I think in long-term care the mistakes are pervasive.

Where do we go from here? The time of my grandmother's stroke provided an important lesson on the basis of which I can suggest what direction we should take. It was not terribly expensive to have grandmother at home. The visiting nurse was helpful. The physician provided care in response to my grandmother's expressed needs. This is not to argue for universal home care or to suggest that lower-cost options are preferable. My reference is to a person who was frightened of hospitals, who was used to running her own home in her own way. It was important for her to be in her own room and with her family. Her *need* was to be at home. The system adapted to *her* needs.

We need to transfer the control of decisions in long-term care to clients. I believe we can build and design systems that can adapt to this need. I think *caring* has to be part of long-term care—caring that is responsive to clients' needs. I believe that by the end of the 1990s, consumers will have control and, as a provider, I will feel better that they have that control. As a funder, I believe that the system will be more effective and efficient. I invite you to capture the vision for the future that I acquired from the experience with my grandmother. It is a vision of a direction in which caring in long-term care will grow out of the consumer's knowledge of the system as well as his or her control of funding in the system.

7

Daily Money Management:
An Emerging Service in Long-Term Care

Kathleen H. Wilber and Leah Buturain

Alice Moyer, seventy-one, was devastated when her husband died suddenly from a heart attack shortly after their fiftieth wedding anniversary. Not only was she overwhelmed by the loss, she was also confronted with a maze of bills and financial records. For the first time in her life she was responsible for managing her finances.

Richard Hernandez, a seventy-nine-year-old widower, was discharged from the hospital two months after suffering a serious stroke. Although he gradually gained strength and appeared to be on the road to a complete recovery, his right side was still partially paralyzed, which limited his ability to walk, write, and feed himself. While the hospital discharge planner had arranged for physical therapy, home health services, and home delivered meals, there was no one to help him tackle the pile of medical bills, insurance forms, and the delinquent mortgage payments and utilities bills that had piled up during his hospitalization.

Sylvia Porter, ninety-one, a retired secretary who had never married, lived in a comfortable retirement community. Her monthly expenses were covered by social security payments, her only source of income. Fiercely

We would like to acknowledge the support of the Administration on Aging and the Randolph Haynes and Dora Haynes Foundation.

self-reliant, she struggled to maintain her independence. But poor vision coupled with episodes of forgetfulness caused her to misplace and misread her bills, which made it difficult for Mrs. Porter to maintain her financial records. Her predicament was discovered by a utility representative when he stopped to inquire about why her payment was delinquent.

Alice Moyer, Richard Hernandez, and Sylvia Porter share a common problem: because of unfortunate circumstances and life crises, they are finding it difficult to pay their bills. Although their needs are different, each would benefit from financial management assistance. Researchers estimate that between 5 and 10 percent of all older adults living in the community require some assistance with basic money management tasks such as bill paying, budgeting, and filling out medical insurance forms.[1] And as the population ages, the number of adults requiring money management services is expected to grow.

This chapter focuses on what money management is and the various approaches used by money management service providers to assist elders who are unable to handle their finances. Our views are based on two studies of money management conducted from 1985 to 1989. The studies catalogued money management services nationwide, examined organizational characteristics of the services, and explored the effectiveness of money management programs to divert elders from guardianship/conservatorship. As part of this research, staff from fifty organizations responded to a written questionnaire, representatives from twenty money management services participated in in-depth phone interviews, and seven on-site studies were conducted. Throughout the chapter, we rely on examples from these studies and particular exemplary programs that are truly the pioneers in money management services. These include the Cathedral Project in Jacksonville, Florida; the Cincinnati Area Senior Services in Cincinnati, Ohio; Kansas Support Services for Elders in Kansas City, Kansas; and Support Services for Elders in San Francisco, California.

"Daily Money Management" (DMM), a term used throughout this chapter, was introduced publicly over a decade ago by a pioneer in the field, Jack McKay, to describe an array of financial services offered by nonprofit social service organizations. DMM refers to a continuum of services directed toward helping frail or at-risk adults manage their financial affairs. The term encompasses numerous tasks and varying levels of intervention aimed at day-to-day financial management activities, such as bill paying and procuring benefits and entitlements. DMM, similar in some respects to the financial planning and investment counseling done by financial institutions such as banks and investment companies, is different in two respects. First, it is geared toward middle- and low-income elders. Second, its day-to-day focus contrasts with investment-based financial planning services that emphasize optimizing investments over the long term.

We begin the discussion of DMM services by examining who needs money management. This is followed by an overview of five services designed to assist elders with money management and the roles and limitations of each type of service. We conclude the chapter with a discussion of what we believe to be the knowledge base and state-of-the-art of money management services and our recommendations for future directions.

WHO NEEDS MONEY MANAGEMENT?

Gerontologists consider money management to be an Instrumental Activity of Daily Living (IADL). Like other IADLs, such as cooking, cleaning, shopping, using the telephone, and taking medication, money management is an activity carried out as part of the daily responsibility of taking care of oneself. Problems managing money may be a harbinger of difficulties in other areas of self-care. Or such problems may mean that the elder is experiencing a temporary crisis that impedes his or her ability to manage personal affairs. As illustrated by Alice Moyer, money management may represent a skill that was never acquired.

Regardless of the origins of the difficulty, money management represents a sensitive area of intervention. The responsibility for managing our money and our assets epitomizes our legal rights of self-determination, autonomy, and independence. In keeping with the rights of older adults to maintain their autonomy, the goal of money management assistance is to support decision making and maximize independence while helping elders pay the rent, balance the checkbook, or file reimbursement forms.

A variety of social, physical, and psychological changes associated with aging may result in the need for money management assistance. These include changing social circumstances, such as widowhood, that may require the surviving spouse to assume new roles. Accidents or illness may result in physical disabilities that impede an elder's ability to undertake the basic mechanics of bill paying. Dementing illnesses, which lead to problems in memory and comprehension may, over time, make it increasingly difficult for elders to manage their financial affairs. Other chronic illnesses, such as arthritis, heart disease, and emphysema, make it difficult to conduct day-to-day activities.

Illness, as well as social losses and isolation, may also contribute to depression resulting in lack of motivation, reduced energy, or disinterest in managing day-to-day affairs. Sensory impairment, particularly visual problems, may make bill paying difficult. Some older persons suffer from a combination of physical and psychological problems that overwhelms their ability to manage their financial affairs. Finally, some elders, particularly those who are socially isolated from friends and family, may find themselves in situations where they are being financially exploited. In addition to depleting the elder's assets, the perpetrator of financial exploitation may seek to further isolate the elder from those who could intervene in the situation.

Although we believe that DMM is a critical service, it has received considerably less attention than have other areas of long-term care. With a few notable exceptions,[2] little has been written on the subject. The small number of research studies that have been conducted include a description of the roles of money management[3] and an investigation of whether or not money management services divert elders from guardianship.[4]

THE DAILY MONEY MANAGEMENT "SOLUTION"

Several different types of assistance are available for elders who need money management assistance. Not surprisingly, for those with considerable assets, a number of fee-for-service or commission-based services exist. Providers of fee-based financial management services include trust officers in the trust departments of banks, accountants, attorneys, stockbrokers, and certified financial planners (CFPs).

While such services appear to work well for those who have sizeable assets, most elders lack the resources required to hire professional financial planners. Therefore, many middle and low-income elders rely on an informal support system comprised of family, friends, and trusted neighbors for help with money management.

Although professional services and informal supports appear to serve the majority of elders who need help, these approaches do not meet the needs of those who are unable to purchase services from financial management establishments in the private market and who do not have friends or family available to offer assistance. Staff from aging-service organizations acknowledge that this gap often is filled by formal providers offering "informal" help with money management. By this we mean that persons who are paid to deliver other types of long-term care services assume responsibility for the bill-paying role as well. For example, the home health aide who visits three times a week, in addition to other tasks, helps see that the bills are paid. Or the case manager, who coordinates long-term care services, recognizing the unmet need, takes on the role of bill-paying assistance.

While such an ad hoc approach may address the problem for specific clients in the short run, it may also create new problems for both the client and the service provider in the long run. In addition to the risk that they will not adequately serve the client's interests, providers who move into the money management role without the authority to do so face issues of liability and role conflict. As providers become aware of this dilemma, they are increasingly looking to the development of formalized DMM services as a financial management solution for elders who are not served by a CFP, friends, or relatives.

What Are DMM Services?

Daily money management is a social service anomaly. While it is neither fish nor fowl, case management nor financial management, it shares similarities with both and is probably best understood as a hybrid. The auspices for DMM services are generally nonprofit social service agencies staffed by social workers and case managers. But unlike social workers and case managers in traditional social services, DMM staff also act as fiduciaries. Because they manage money for clients, DMM staff must work closely with private, for-profit entities, such as banks and savings and loans, to accomplish their work. Thus, the DMM staff need to be able to interact with the network of social and health-service providers as well as the banking and financial community. DMM services run the gamut from short-term help with education and organizing to long-term hands-on assistance with bill paying. In many instances, DMM staff assist clients who retain legal authority to make all of their own financial decisions. In some situations, however, a DMM agency actually assumes the legal responsibility for client assets. DMM services may be found as part of case management services, senior centers, hospitals, and other community-based service system providers.[5] They may also be offered as "free standing" services by agencies whose sole mission is to provide money management assistance.

A CONCEPTUAL OVERVIEW OF DMM SERVICES

As we began to study DMM, we were struck by the lack of uniformity between programs. Because there were no blueprints and few program models, DMM services often developed in an ad hoc fashion as client needs were recognized. The result was a variety of approaches to organizing and delivering DMM services. In order to clarify what DMM services actually do, we found it useful to catalog and conceptually organize the services along a continuum.

This continuum, as shown in Figure 1, identifies five distinct roles

FIGURE 1
DAILY MONEY MANAGEMENT (DMM)

CONTINUUM OF SERVICES

Agency's Role:	Advising & Advocating	
Services Provided:	• Information & Referral (I&R) • Public Benefits Advocacy	ADVANCE PLANNING: • Durable Power of Attorney for Health Care (DPHAC) • Wills • Burial Plans
Client's Role:	Consumer	

Agency's Role:	Planning & Assisting
Services Provided:	• Budgeting • Bill Paying Assistance • Direct Deposit • Insurance Billing
Client's Role:	Bill Payer

FIGURE 1 (cont.)

DAILY MONEY MANAGEMENT (DMM)

CONTINUUM OF SERVICES

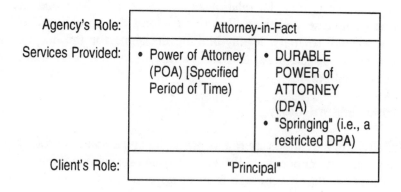

Agency's Role:	Attorney-in-Fact	
Services Provided:	• Power of Attorney (POA) [Specified Period of Time)	• DURABLE POWER of ATTORNEY (DPA) • "Springing" (i.e., a restricted DPA)
Client's Role:	"Principal"	

Agency's Role:	Representative Payee	Guardian/Conservator
Services Provided:	• Representative Payee	• Guardianship (conservatorship) a. Person Only b. Estate Only c. Person and Estate
Client's Role:	Claimant Beneficiary	Ward Conservatee

carried out by DMM services. These are (a) advising and advocacy, (b) planning and assisting, (c) "attorney-in-fact," (d) representative or substitute payee, and, (3) guardian or conservator. Although not all organizations take on all five of the roles, these functions together constitute the continuum of DMM services. The continuum begins with cell one, which shows the agency role as one of advising and advocating. In this capacity, the agency acts as educator and information provider, and the recipient of services operates as autonomous consumer. Moving from left to right across the continuum and vertically down the page, each cell represents greater legal intervention. As the relationship between the provider and recipient becomes more formalized, greater accountability and legal responsibility is required on the part of the agency. Another way of saying this is that the relationship between the client and the agency is one of inverse power. As we move along the continuum, the power of the agency to make legally-binding decisions for the client increases. The roles, responsibilities, and legal authority of providers and recipients are discussed below.

Advising and Advocacy

The advising and advocacy role is primarily an educational role that serves to enhance the capacity of the elder to manage with minimal assistance. A capacity-building approach is most appropriate for someone like Alice Moyer, the recent widow discussed in the case example above, who, prior to her husband's death, had never needed to manage her finances. In order that she may assume responsibility for her finances, Mrs. Moyer needs education, including instructions on how to organize her finances, balance her checkbook, and master the mechanics of banking procedures. Organizing her finances may include arranging for direct-deposit banking and automatic bill-paying services. She may wish to learn about benefits and entitlements, including the terms of her husband's will and retirement income, such as pension arrangements and social security. And, if needed, the DMM staff can help ensure that she is receiving all the benefits to which she is entitled. In addition, Mrs. Moyer may want to plan for her future by working with the money manager to develop advance directives that spell out her preferences in the event that she loses the capacity to make decisions for herself. She may also work with the DMM program staff to ensure that her burial plans and will are in order.

Mrs. Moyer's relationship to the provider organization is one of consumer. She employs an expert to help her develop necessary skills, but retains legal authority to make all decisions regarding her finances and to determine what she wants to learn and how long the relationship continues. If Mrs. Moyer's finances are not unduly complicated, we would expect the intervention to be short-term. In all likelihood, two or three sessions should be sufficient time for Mrs. Moyer to acquire money-management skills.

Planning and Assistance

The role of planning and assisting is the one most frequently associated with money-management services. The major differences between this role and the advising and advocacy role is that planning and assisting most often involves direct, hands-on help with bill paying rather than the "how-to" instruction associated with the advising and advocacy role. Elders who require planning and assistance, in general, require more help for an extended period of time—much longer than do those who require advising and advocacy. In the planning and assisting capacity, the agency typically provides ongoing long-term support to a client rather than a brief instructional intervention.

Elders who are served tend to be more functionally dependent on the service agency to assist with money-management activities and often provide other services as well. Despite these functional dependencies, we think that it is important to recognize that, in this role, as well as in the advising and advocacy role, all decision making resides with the client. Rather than appropriating the bill paying or other DMM functions, the money manager is expected to support clients' decisions and to help clients execute their decisions. Therefore, DMM staff presume that clients are competent to make decisions unless there is consistent evidence of incapacity, in which case planning and assisting is not the appropriate intervention. Daily money-management roles in situations where clients lack decisional capacity are discussed below.

As with the advising and advocacy role, client education may be provided here as well. Generally, however, providers serving in this role do more than educate. They provide assistance with a variety of banking and bill-paying activities. This role is inappropriate for functionally dependent clients (such as Richard Hernandez), who can participate in bill-paying activities if they receive adequate guidance and monitoring. Tasks undertaken by the money manager in the planning and assistance role include: helping the client to organize bills, fill out Medicare forms, complete insurance claims, and collect financial records; ongoing budgeting; banking; and advocacy, including arranging for benefits as well as other in-home and community-based long-term care services.

Paperwork and the processing of forms can easily overwhelm an older person who suffers from visual problems or money deficits. Therefore, barring an immediate crisis, the first step for a DMM staff member serving in the planning and assistance role is to conduct an assessment. Basic organization of bills and assets is essential to develop an accurate picture of the client's financial state. In addition to determining debts and available assets, such an assessment can be used to identify and address areas that require immediate attention.

In cases of long-term financial neglect, which are by no means rare in DMM, organizing bills and records may prove quite challenging. Situations where bill-paying activities have been ignored for long periods of time may take months to sort out. To address the problem of sorting out complex paperwork, some programs create a system using expandable files, while others have clients and visitors put all paper in a large mailbox placed inside the door. After the money manager has assessed the situation and dealt with immediate concerns, the next step is to develop a budget that estimates how money will be expended in an average month. Although DMM does not typically involve investment counseling, some long-term planning may be necessary. For example, clients may be unaware that they have assets such as government bonds or certificates of deposit. The money manager and the client may decide how to handle such assets or, in some cases, the money manager will refer the client to an appropriate financial planner. Budgeting is also used to identify tasks that must be completed weekly, monthly, quarterly, and annually.

Once the client's records have been organized and a budget has been developed, ongoing maintenance activities are the primary focus. Maintenance activities may include processing checks to pay bills; balancing bank statements; and posting deposits, withdrawals, and financial records. If the clients receive these papers in their home, these numbers are posted, or documented in their checkbook. If the bills come to the agency, they are posted in the ledger books.

Bill-paying help may take several forms. The client may make out checks while the staff person provides instruction. The client may prepare the check for review by the DMM staff member, who ensures that the work is correct. Most commonly, the DMM staff member completes the check for the client to sign. When this approach is used, care must be taken to ensure that the client understands the nature of the expenditure and what is being signed.

Banking constitutes a third area of services in the planning-and-assisting role. The money manager may represent the client at the bank by opening an account or changing the type of account, close or consolidate other bank accounts, arrange for a bank power of attorney, or secure a safety-deposit box. The Cathedral Project in Jacksonville, Florida, and Cincinnati Area Senior Services, in Ohio, both in operation, are examples of DMM banking services. Both respond to the needs that many elders have for assistance with banking and transportation by generating checks and running banking errands for clients. However, their approach, which requires staff to conduct banking business on behalf of the elders, is not feasible for agencies that have policies prohibiting staff from handling cash. In such situations, meeting the banking needs of clients becomes a greater challenge. In general, programs tend either to assist clients in their homes and accompany them to the bank, or to have the bills sent to the agency to be processed there. Banking services, which greatly reduce the need for visits to the bank, such as direct-deposit banking and automatic bill paying may also be arranged.

The final area discussed in this section is similar to advocacy in that it involves securing benefits and linking clients to other needed services. Indeed, this is a function that cuts across all of the DMM roles listed in Figure 1. However, the need to link clients with other services is most likely to be encountered in the planning-and-assisting role. DMM clients, such as Mr. Hernandez, who suffer from chronic physical, cognitive, or sensory impairments, often require long-term care services in addition to money management. If other needs are identified, DMM staff may serve as service coordinators, linking the client with other services.

We think that it is important to recognize that such a coordinating role may contribute to problems with respect to conflict of interest. Although participation in a DMM program is voluntary and clients are free to terminate at any point, the role of money manager involves some degree of actual or perceived control over the client's finances. Therefore, DMM program staff must be aware of and sensitive to who benefits from services purchased by the client. Conflicts are especially apparent when referrals are made to other services within the DMM organization. Because the potential for conflict of interest is always present when dealing with money, DMM programs need to maintain policies that avoid real or perceived conflict of interest, and implement mechanisms to ensure that clients' interests are safeguarded. Such procedures should at minimum include thorough documentation of all transactions and referrals, including client consent forms indicating that procedures have been presented to clients in straightforward terms and signed and dated by the client.

Some agencies create ad hoc committees that make decisions for referrals on a case-by-case basis. In addition, some agencies protect themselves from possible charges of conflict of interest by referring their clients to at least three different professionals and letting the client make the selection. For example, a referral to an attorney might be made to the local bar association or a list of attorneys provided with the disclaimer that the individuals are not endorsed. However, clients needing assistance may press the money manager for a recommendation. DMM providers acknowledge that in most cases, the person handing the client a list will be asked, "Which one would you recommend?" Regardless of the approach, the problem of referrals outside of the agency remain a challenging and unresolved issue.

In addition to serving as a broker for other professionals, DMM staff also benefit clients by linking them to volunteers who provide such valuable assistance as tax preparation or attorneys who offer pro bono* work.

Bill-Paying Assistance

Some DMM services stop in cell two of the continuum. There is nothing wrong with limiting services to these two roles as long as the agency is explicit about what is provided. For example, if an agency is not going to handle cash or take any legal responsibility, it might be advisable to call the program Bill-Paying Assistance instead of DMM. Regardless of what is offered, a clear statement of the services helps potential consumers understand what is available and helps other agencies avoid inappropriate referrals. In addition, clear language about the services that are and are not offered may help an agency limit its liability. For example, an agency that offers only bill-paying assistance is not likely to encounter problems because it was expected to provide financial planning.

"Attorney-in-Fact"

Up to this point we have discussed approaches that are designed to enhance rather than to replace an elder's decision-making capacity in financial management. We turn now to powers-of-attorney (POA). A POA is an arrangement whereby an elder delegates authority to make decisions to another individual or to an organizational entity. POA services are those for which the agency takes legal responsibility for handling the finances of a person who has the capacity to sign a legal document and gives legal authority to the agency to carry out stipulated or general activities. In this capacity, a DMM organization serves in the role of "attorney-in-fact." Whereas the first role, advising and advocacy, was viewed as capacity-building, and the second role planning and assistance, involved enabling support, a POA involves the transfer of responsibility to another. The elder, referred to in this agreement as "the principal," legally delegates authority to another individual or in an organizational entity, such as a DMM service, termed the "attorney-in-fact." Once designated as

---

*legal assistance that is free of charge as a public service

attorney-in-fact, the money manager is given authority to act on behalf of the elder in specified areas.

The scope of legal and financial authority transferred from the principal to the attorney-in-fact may be very broad. Or, a POA may consist of a specific activity or transaction, such as selling a car. Although authority is delegated to another, a POA may be revoked by the principal at any time. If it is not revoked, a POA remains in effect as long as the principal retains legal capacity to make decisions. (The area of legal capacity will be discussed more extensively below.) A POA agreement is automatically revoked if the principal loses capacity.

Mr. Hernandez might make use of a power-of-attorney initially while he is recovering from his stroke. If his health improves and he is able to regain use of his right side through therapy, he may be able to do more on his own. In light of the problems he faces at discharge (i.e., multiple bills and impaired mobility), he may decide to sign a limited POA giving the money manager authority to sign checks for a certain period of time. The money manager should also apply for a specific POA with Mr. Hernandez's bank to ensure that he has the bank's cooperation in conducting banking for Mr. Hernandez.

In addition to a general POA, several types of advance directives utilizing powers-of-attorney are of potential use for DMM participants. A durable power-of-attorney (DPA) is similar to a general power-of-attorney in that it authorizes transfer of authority under specified conditions. It differs, however, in that it is binding even after the elder has lost the cognitive capacity to execute agreements. Thus, elders who might select this option would be those who wanted assurance that an individual or organization of their choice would manage their affairs in the event of lost capacity.

In contrast to Mr. Hernandez, Alice Moyer does not think that she needs a power-of-attorney arrangement currently. However, she has learned through her participation in a DMM program that it is possible that she may need more help in the future. She decides that it is prudent to spell out financial and health-care decisions so that her wishes are carried out in the event that she becomes incapacitated. Her state allows for a durable power of attorney (DPA) with a springing mechanism (sometimes referred to as a Springing DPA), which enables a power-of-attorney to be activated by pre-specified criteria (e.g., if she were determined to be decisionally incapacitated by two qualified professionals). She realizes that once enacted in accordance with the stipulated criteria, she cannot revoke the Springing DPA.

In addition to financial management, DPAs are increasingly used as advance directives for health-care decisions. In the state of California, for example, an elder can execute a durable-power-of-attorney-for-health-care (DPAHC) that nominates a decision maker in the event that the principal loses the capacity to make health-care decisions as a result of illness or accident. Mrs. Moyer signs a DPAHC nominating a trusted friend to serve as the "attorney-in-fact" because she is confident the friend will make decisions in accordance with her expressed wishes and her values.

Because the basic philosophy of DMM is to empower clients and to support the decisions they make, providing assistance with advance directives is a critical component of many DMM programs. But, it is important that DMM agencies ensure that all clients executing a POA or an advance directive understand what they are agreeing to and the consequences of their decisions. In San Francisco, in order to confirm that the client comprehends the POA agreement or the DPA, Support Services for Elders (SSE) requires their staff to check the client's understanding and comprehension of the agreement during three separate visits. During each visit, DMM staff attempt to ascertain if the client understands the authority that is being transferred to the DMM agency. If the person seems confused or changes his or her mind, a case conference results to determine the course of action.

Unfortunately, elders are often referred to DMM programs after they no longer have the cognitive capacity to make financial decisions. In cases where the principal lacks the capacity to make informed decisions, the POA is invalid. If the elder requires help and is lacking the capacity to execute agreements, substituted judgment in the form of a surrogate decision maker may be used. The most common types of substituted judgment, representative payee and guardianship, are discussed below.

Representative Payee

Each of the approaches discussed so far requires that the elder consent to participate in a DMM service or agree to delegate authority to the DMM organization. But what happens if it appears that the elder needs help and there is strong evidence that he or she is decisionally incapacitated? Representative payeeship is one mechanism that may be used in such circumstances. Also known as substitute payee, representative payees have authority over government benefits, such as Social Security and Supplemental Security Income. The Social Security Administration (SSA) grants this authority when it has evidence that the elder does not have the capacity to handle funds. The SSA may require that a representative payeeship, whether or not the elder—termed the beneficiary here and initially referred to as the claimant by SSA—agrees to relinquish authority.

Some agencies, however, will only take over a representative payeeship for beneficiaries who voluntarily consent to participate.

Agencies cannot charge a fee for the representative payeeship service, which inhibits the willingness of many DMMs to provide this service. However, forty agencies that wish to provide primarily the representative payeeship service have turned to the volunteer representative payee program developed by Legal Counsel for the Elderly (LCE), a division of the American Association of Retired Persons (AARP) for sponsorship. The LCE recruits volunteers by sending letters to AARP members in a service area, provides training, then receives the monthly cancelled checks and bank statements to ensure that the beneficiaries' money is being handled responsibly.[6]

Sylvia Porter might benefit from a representative payee program if it were determined that she lacked the decisional capacity to participate in the money management areas discussed earlier. By decisional incapacity, we mean that she lacks the ability to understand the consequences of her actions. It is possible that she would welcome assistance from a surrogate who could handle her finances. On the other hand, given her sense of independence, she may not at all be pleased by such an arrangement, in which case a decision would have to be made that balanced the risk she faces if she continues unassisted and her cognitive capacity to understand that risk. If she has the capacity to understand what she is refusing and the consequences of her refusal, then the appointment of a surrogate decision maker is inappropriate. If, however, she lacks the capacity to comprehend her situation, then a representative payee, or even a guardianship, may be appropriate.

The assessment of capacity is difficult at best. For representative payee programs, the evidence of incapacity to manage public entitlements must come from a physician who has examined the patient within the last twelve months. The physician signs a government form stating that the person in question does not have the capacity to handle his or her finances on grounds of "mental" and/or "physical" impairments. Controversy exists over the adequacy of this requirement. The representative payeeship program is also faulted because of lack of oversight and standards for the person serving as representative payee. The last several years have witnessed a number of lawsuits brought against the SSA for failure to safeguard those who require a representative payee.

Guardianship/Conservatorship

Guardianship, or conservatorship, as it is called in some states, is like representative payeeship in that it involves the appointment of a surrogate decision maker to serve an individual who lacks the capacity to manage his or her financial affairs. It differs from representative payee in that it is determined by court order. It is also broader, encompassing all sources of income and often involving control of personal as well as financial decisions. Under a guardianship arrangement, an individual or an organizational entity (called the guardian or conservator) manages the affairs of another (called the ward or conservatee). Guardianship or conservatorship may involve managing the estate (the property, income, and assets of the ward) and/or the person (ensure that the ward's basic personal needs are met). Most often, guardians are appointed to manage both the estate and the person. Although the court may limit the guardian's responsibility to particular areas, usually the guardian is granted broad authority to make decisions regarding all aspects of the ward's life. Therefore, in addition to handling the ward's finances, the guardian is responsible for determining where the ward lives, authorizing medical treatment, and making personal decisions as though a parent were making them on behalf of a minor.

It is estimated that more than 500,000 persons nationwide have been appointed to guardianships. The average age of wards is eighty, and more than half reside in nursing homes.[7] Although the purpose of guardianship is to safeguard dependent persons who may otherwise be vulnerable to mistreatment, exploitation, and neglect, a number of problems have been identified. Concerns include the tendency of guardianship proceedings to be rubber-stamped resulting in a high percentage of petitions leading to appointment. Often, elders are not represented by an attorney and some are not even present during court proceedings. In addition, the actual time spent in the courtroom may be very brief. Because of the perfunctory nature of many guardianship hearings and the tendency of such proceedings to result in appointment to guardianship, there is concern that some elders who become wards do not require such a restrictive intervention. For example, while Mrs. S. was in the hospital undergoing surgery, a neighbor petitioned the court for guardianship stating that Mrs. S. was incompetent to manage her affairs. Although the court claimed to have made an effort to reach her, Mrs. S. was not notified that she had been appointed to guardianship, and that her guardian had sold her home and its contents "to pay for her medical care." Upon discharge from the hospital Mrs. S. was notified by her court-appointed guardian that arrangements had been made for her to enter a nursing home. Mrs. S. protested and demanded a court hearing. The judge refused to hear her case, stating that because she had been declared incompetent she had no legal right to petition the court.

To address such problems, legal scholars and advocates for the elderly have promoted limited guardianships that would remain in effect for a designated period of time. In addition, critics have protested that guardianship standards and regulations are inadequate. And there is concern about the lack of judicial oversight of guardians.[8]

Although the role of the guardian involves financial management, controversy exists over whether guardianship constitutes the final service of the DMM continuum, or whether DMM services exist to avoid appointment to guardianship. We believe that guardianship is an essential service that should be included in a DMM service continuum. However, we also realize that a number of factors influence whether or not a DMM agency includes guardianship as one of its basic services. DMM agencies deciding whether or not to include guardianship as one of their services must consider the existing resources and service options available to clients, especially whether or not gaps exist in guardianship services. Some communities have adequate public and private guardianship services available for the clients who need them. In other communities such services are difficult to obtain.

DMM agencies can serve in several guardianship capacities. They can take on the money-management role or management of the estate for guardians who serve in the role of both person and estate. This service is particularly useful for family caregivers who could benefit from support with financial matters. DMM programs can also serve as guardian for elders who have been money-management clients. Finally, DMM services may provide guardianship services to elders who cannot afford to pay for private guardians. This role is becoming increasingly important in communities where public guardian programs are unavailable or underfunded.

Practically speaking, the leadership of each DMM service makes the decision on whether to serve in the role of guardian depend on a host of factors, including but not limited to, existing resources in the community, state legislation, liability issues, the agency's insurance coverage, and, probably most important, its values and philosophical perpsective on guardianship. Some providers feel that they can serve clients better by offering the full continuum of services, thus being available regardless of what.is needed. One DMM director commented, "I will not accept clients who need a guardianship at the outset. However, if any of my clients whom I have served over increasing degrees of dependency becomes incapacitated, I will not turn my back on them in their greatest time of need." Others argue that their mission is to avoid guardianship for their clients. Believing that to petition for guardianship is to petition against the client, they are unwilling to take the position of attempting to prove that a client lacks the capacity to make decisions.

Some DMM providers attempt to avoid the conflict of testifying that a client lacks the capacity to manage by avoiding the role of petitioner for guardianship. Such agencies will serve as guardians if two criteria are met: first, the prospective ward must be a client at the time the petition is filed; second, the petition itself must be filed by someone outside of the agency.

DAILY MONEY MANAGEMENT: STATE OF THE ART

The last decade has witnessed a growing recognition of the need for DMM coupled with the development of a scattered number of programs nationwide. Other activities include the first DMM conference, which was held in Pasadena, California,[9] the development of a nationwide core of volunteers, under the auspices of American Association for Retired Persons' Legal Counsel for the Elderly to serve as representative payees, and the funding of several DMM research and demonstration projects by the Administration on Aging. Despite these developments, DMM is programmatically still in its infancy and a number of localities remain without such services. Yet, from all evidence the need for DMM services will grow. Demographers tell us that we are living longer and that our family structures are changing. Family caregivers are providing the majority of services for frail elderly relatives. And we are seeing increasingly complex and sophisticated financial transactions. While some agencies have been willing to deal with the need for money management by balancing checkbooks "unofficially," the threat of liability has forced the hand of many agency directors and their boards either to forbid informal assistance or to develop policies and procedures to provide the service formally.

During the short time period that innovators have been experimenting with money management services, a number of valuable lessons have been learned. This final section discusses what we have learned and where we should go from here.

What Do We Know About DMM Service Delivery?

First, DMM services should be formalized. Formalization requires the development of policies and procedures that safeguard both the providers and the clients. An "informal" or "backroom" approach to services only serves to "tempt fate" by increasing the risk for both parties. The untrained person may expend the elder's resources inappropriately or ineffectively, whereupon he or she is vulnerable to accusations of misuse of funds.

Second, we know or at least strongly suspect that DMM services work best when they are able to garner strong community support. DMM clients are likely to need additional services from other long-term care providers. Therefore, services are most effective when linkages are arranged with other long-term care services. Support Services for Elders (SSE), for example, has a Technical Advisory Committee (TAC) comprised of fifty-two agencies serving older adults in the San Francisco area. This advisory committee is divided into five subcommittees: banking, real estate and investment, legal, funding, social services, and public relations. The TAC reports to the board of directors. The members are active in developing referrals and educating the community about SSE's services. Involving as many community agencies as possible in the planning stages increases the effectiveness of the service, helps community members feel invested, and enables the program to be built as a coalition in spirit as well as in practice.

Third, the development of community linkages and clarification of staff roles are also important because of potential overlap between DMM activities and other service areas. DMM generally works best in conjunction with case management, either as an integral part with the same agency or working in close cooperation with case managers from other agencies. For example, the case manager may arrange for in-home services or assist in placing the client in a nursing facility but may turn to the money manager to assist the client in creating DPAHC, or a DPA for Assets Management, or arranging for a burial plan and signing of an agreement. While case management is important to support DMM services, there is often a reciprocal information flow. Because knowledge about DMM has only recently been formulated, case managers may be unaware of finance-related questions to ask during an initial case assessment. For example, in order to document the need in communities where no DMM services exist and in order to make appropriate referrals when DMM services are present, case managers need to ask the client such questions as: Who pays the bills? Do you have a DPAHC? Do you have a will? Do you have a burial plan?

Fourth, we are increasingly aware that the development and implementation of DMM services offer numerous and often formidable challenges to providers. DMM staff have shared with us such start-up difficulties as recruiting and bonding staff who have the dual competencies of a client-centered social service perspective and financial management expertise. And, if the number of providers who have abandoned DMM services is any indication, problems do not end with implementation. Sustaining DMM services is also difficult. DMM agencies are concerned, and justifiably so, about acquiring adequate liability coverage for other professional staff, volunteers, and clients. Even if an insurance company is willing to insure, e.g., for "loss of funds," it is still difficult to find and pay for "third-party insurance. Since, as attorneys are quick to point out, "anyone can sue for anything," an agency may have to hire legal services to defend itself. Given the budget constraints of nonprofits, this prospect, although unlikely, can still prove daunting. DMM programs face the ongoing problem of generating sufficient fee-for-service clients to offset some of the expenses for this labor-intensive service. Indeed, many of the programs are still not charging fees. Because of the meaning of money in our culture[10] and because financial services are both personal and privileged information, DMM services may engender greater resistance than more concrete services, such as meals, transportation, or home health.

Fifth, although the area of client targeting and the question of who requires which type of service needs to be explored further, we believe that the continuum of services outlined in figure 1 represents distinct services. Clients may require different services at different points in time; however, we do not believe that these services generally substitute for each other. For example, when we examined the ability of DMM to divert elders from guardianship, we were hopeful that the less restrictive DMM services would, in fact, reduce the rates of guardianship in our samples. Two studies that examined this area led to the same outcome: rates of guardianship were not changed by participation in less restrictive DMM roles.[11]

Sixth, based on our work with protective service clients, we have also come, reluctantly, to the conclusion that DMM services are no panacea. Unfortunately, however, it has been our experience that some communities fail to set realistic goals for what these services can and cannot accomplish. Like most long-term care services, those of DMM do not provide ready solutions for such intractable issues as dangerously self-neglecting elders or victims of exploitation who refuse intervention. Failure to manage one's money can lead to severe immediate repercussions. But money management problems can also represent less visible underlying issues. In some situations, problems handling finances can be a symptom of dementing illnesses. In other circumstances, money management problems represent lifelong patterns of neglect and abdication of responsibility resulting from such problems as mental disorders and substance abuse. Still in others, money management troubles can indicate a temporary crisis. Although DMM services have much to offer elders like Alice Moyer, Richard Hernandez, and Sylvia Porter, they are not a cure-all for older persons who suffer from neglect or exploitation or who place themselves at risk because they are unwilling or unable to provide adequately for their basic needs. DMM services should be part of the array of long-term care services available to impaired elders. But because many elders who require DMM services have multiple impairments that compound their need for assistance, DMM can only provide part of the solution.

Finally, DMM services involve some risk on the part of the provider; and no matter how careful the provider is in safeguarding the interests of all the parties involved, a modicum of paranoia in the area of liability is justified. Insurance companies are reluctant to insure DMM services, or when they do agree to write a policy a large charge is added to the agency's regular coverage because, as one provider noted, "there is greater risk for someone who manages money than someone who cleans the house." But practically speaking, anytime someone goes into a person's home, especially if the client is cognitively impaired or has a mental disorder, there is always the threat of being accused of misappropriation of money. In many instances such complaints result from the client's illness. Nevertheless, the possibility of financial exploitation must be recognized. Access to a checkbook or to a bank account may offer the temptation to exploit the situation, and there are cases where workers have simply helped themselves. We are aware of a recent incident where a money manager with nine years of service was caught embezzling money from a wealthy client. Staff who had perceived him to be a caring and competent co-worker felt betrayed when they realized that he had been, throughout his tenure, a compulsive gambler.

Another area of potential risk that DMM providers should consider and plan for is the desire of clients to try to compensate the professional's kind and competent assistance by offering gifts or naming the money manager in their will. Some clients develop affectionate bonds with their money managers, whom they may consider as surrogate family. As difficult as it may be, we recommend that all significant gifts and all gifts of money be graciously refused. Given clients' vulnerability and the power inherent in the relationship, the gift may be considered given under "undue influence." Thus, a third party could accuse the worker of being solicitous and winning the favor of the elder in order to take advantage of the client's gratitude. Further, if a client expresses interest in including the DMM agency in his or her will, the agency is advised to refer the client to independent legal counsel to avoid the possibility of "undue influence."

These examples indicate the risk inherent in providing services that deal with money. But as one executive director remarked, "I could wait until everything looked safe, but meanwhile clients would be evicted, exploited, and prematurely placed in nursing homes using state dollars unnecessarily. I'd rather take the risk and do the best job possible. Even a few additional months of autonomy make it worth my effort."

WHERE DO WE GO FROM HERE?

The last decade has witnessed increasing recognition of the need for DMM services, and we have learned a great deal from the successes and failures of money management programs. But with a few notable exceptions, we have not had much success translating that knowledge into effective DMM programs. Often gerontology and social work majors lack basic training in finance and in related legal issues. If the money manager does not have the expertise, the board of directors and/or technical advisory group must.

Despite the progress in delivering DMM services, as illustrated by the exemplar services discussed throughout this chapter, there still is little information available on DMM. To name just one of the many knowledge deficits, there is neither any written information explaining additional coverage that may be helpful for agencies providing DMM, nor is there anything written to inform insurance companies about the potential risks and responsibilities of this service. Although it is standard to call for further research, we feel that such a recommendation is more than justified. At a minimum, we need to know the effectiveness of various approaches and structures and the outcomes of DMM services. We also need to do more to identify problem areas and effective "best practices" strategies. With the lessons learned by pioneer DMM programs, there is new opportunity for programs to avoid "recreating the wheel" and to be forewarned about the challenging yet laborious nature of these services.

At the same time, the rewarding stories of those whose autonomy was preserved and even recovered offers incentives to fill the existing service gap with creative, workable programs. When concerns about dishonesty, greed, and litigious threats arise, it is helpful to remember a bank vice-president's recent words: "The bottom line is, once your agencies assess the risk, are they willing to implement policies and actions to minimize the risks they're taking?" It is no small coincidence that three of the longstanding programs are those which have operated on the trust of the local community to provide these services "in good faith" while doing the necessary documentation and related homework. Many of the program directors possess a certain style of leadership that looks the beast straight in the eye as if to say, "We know you could attack, but we're prepared and we mean business." Ultimately, it is the work of each community to provide such leadership in order to create services that meet the needs of its citizens.

NOTES

1. National Center for Health Statistics, *Advanced Data: Aging in the Eighties.* No. 133, 1987; R. I. Stone and C. M. Murtaugh, "The Elderly Population with Chronic Functional Disability: Implications for Home Care Eligibility," *The Gerontologist* 30 (1990):491–502.

2. F. L. Feldman (ed.), *Daily Money Management: State of the Art.* Conference Proceedings: Senior Care Network, Pasadena, Calif.: Huntington Memorial Hospital, 1990; J. McKay, "Protective Services," *Generations* 3 (1984):10–13.

3. L. Buturain, "National Survey of Daily Money Management Programs." Unpublished manuscript, 1988.

4. K. H. Wilbur, "Evaluation of Guardianship/Conservatorship and Institutionalizaton Diversion National Demonstration Project." Final Report to the Adminstration on Aging, 1988. See also her "Characteristics of Elders Who Benefit From Money Management Services." Final Report to the Haynes Foundation, 1989.

5. Buturain, "Daily Money Management."

6. J. Hortum, "Representative Payeeship: AARP Models," in Feldman (ed.) *Daily Money Management.* Also T. Jones, 1990 (personal communication) American Association of Retired Persons, Legal Council for the Elderly, Washington, D.C.

7. U.S. House of Representatives, Select Committee on Aging. *Abuses in Guardianship of the Elderly and Infirm: A National Disgrace.* Washington, D.C.: U.S. Government Printing Office, 1987. C. Flemming and E. Dejowski, *Financial Management Services: State-of-the-Art.* Human Resources Administration of the City of New York—Project Focus (October 1982). U.S. House of Representatives, Select Committee on Aging. *Abuses in Guardianship.*

8. W. G. Bell, W. Schmidt, and K. Miller, "Public Guardianship and the Elderly: Findings from a National Study," *The Gerontologist* 21 (1981):194–201. See also J. H. Pickering, "Judicial Practices in Guardianship Proceedings." Statement to the U.S. House of Representatives Select Committee on Aging. Washington, D.C.: U.S. Government Printing Office, 1987; J. J. Regan, "Protective Services for the Elderly: Benefit or Threat." In J. I. Kosberg (ed.) *Abuse and Maltreatment of the Elderly: Causes and Interventions* (Boston: PSG, Inc., 1983), pp. 279–291; W. C. Schmidt, K. S. Miller, W. G. Bell, and B. E. New, *Public Guardianship and the Elderly* (Cambridge, Mass.: Ballinger Publishing Company, 1981); U.S. House of Representatives, Select Committee on Aging. *Abuses in Guardianship;* and U.S. Senate, Special Committee on Aging. *Surrogate Decisionmaking for Adults: Model Standards to Ensure Quality*

Guardianship and Representative Payeeship Services (Washington, D.C.: U.S. Government Printing Office, 1988).

    9. Feldman (ed.), *Daily Money Management.*

    10. Feldman, "Meanings of Money and the Elderly," in Feldman (ed.) *Daily Money Management.*

    11. Wilber, "Evaluation of Guardianship" and "Characteristics of Elders."

REFERENCES

"A Special Report: Guardians of the Elderly." Associated Press, (1987).

Bell, W. G., W. Schmidt, and K. Miller. "Public Guardianship and the Elderly: Findings From a National Study." *The Gerontologist* 21 (1981):194–202.

Buturain, L. "National Survey of Daily Money Management Programs." Unpublished manuscript, 1988.

Feldman, F. L. *Daily Money Management: State of the Aert.* Conference Proceedings: Senior Care Network, Pasadena, Calif.: Huntington Memorial Hospital, 1990.

———. "Meanings of Money and the Elderly." In F. L. Feldman (ed.) *Daily Money Management: State of the Art.* Conference Proceedings. Senior Care Network, Pasadena, Calif.: Huntington Memorial Hospital, 1990.

Flemming, C., and E. Dejowski. *Financial Management Services: State-of-the-Art.* Human Resources Administration of the City of New York —Project Focus. (October 1982).

Friedman, L., and M. Savage. "Taking Care: The Law of Conservatorship in California." *Southern California Law Review* (1988).

Grant, D. "Community-Based Money Management Services: The Missing In-Home Supportive Service Strategy Needed to Preserve Independence." Washington, D.C.: American Association of Retired Persons (December 1987).

Heller, J. L. *Planning Ahead: The Complete Manual on State Surrogate Financial Management Legislation.* Washington, D.C.: American Association of Retired Persons, 1989.

Hortum, J. "Representative Payeeship: AARP Models." In F. L. Feldman (ed.) *Daily Money Management: State of the Art.* Conference Proceedings: Senior Care Network, Pasadena, Calif.: Huntington Memorial Hospital, 1990.

McKay, J. "Protective Services." *Generations* 3 (1984):10–13.

Morrissey, M. "Guardians Ad Litem: An Educational Program in Virginia." *The Gerontologist* 22 (1982):301–304.

National Center for Health Statistics. *Advanced Data: Aging in the Eighties,* No. 133.

Pickering, J. H. "Judicial Practices in Guardianship Proceedings." Statement to the U.S. House of Representatives, Select Committee on Aging. Washington, D.C.: U.S. Government Printing Office, 1987.

Regan, J. J. "Protective Services for the Elderly: Benefit or Threat." In J. I. Kosberg (ed.) *Abuses and Maltreatment of the Elderly: Causes and Interventions.* Mass.: PSG, Inc., 1983, pp. 279–291.

Schmidt, W. C., K. S. Miller, W. G. Bell, and B. E. New. *Public Guardianship and the Elderly.* Cambridge, Mass.: Ballinger Publishing Company, 1981.

Steinberg, R. M. *Alternative Approaches to Conservatorship and Protection of Older Adults Referred to the Public Guardian.* Los Angeles, Calif.: Andrus Gerontology Center, 1985.

Stone, R. I., and C. M. Murtaugh. "The Elderly Population with Chronic Functional Disability: Implications for Home Care Eligibility." *The Gerontologist* 30 (1990):491–502.

U.S. House of Representatives, Select Committee on Aging. *Abuses in Guardianship of the Elderly and Infirm: A National Disgrace.* Washington, D.C.: U.S. Government Printing Office, 1987.

U.S. Senate, Special Committee on Aging. *Surrogate Decisionmaking for Adults: Model Standards to Ensure Quality Guardianship and Representative Payeeship Services.* Washington, D.C.: U.S. Government Printing Office, 1988.

White, M. "Daily Money Management: A Brief Overview." In F. L. Feldman (ed.) *Daily Money Management: State of the Art.* Conference Proceedings: Senior Care Network, Pasadena, Calif.: Huntington Memorial Hospital, 1990.

Wilber, K. H. "Evaluation of Guardianship/Conservatorship and Institutionalization Diversion National Demonstration Project." Final Report to the Administration on Aging, 1988.

———. "Characteristics of Elders Who Benefit from Money Management Services." Final Report to the Haynes Foundation. 1989.

———. "Material Abuse of the Elderly: When Is Guardianship a Solution?" *Journal of Elder Abuse and Neglect* 2 (1990): 89–104.

8

The Noncompliant Elderly

Mary Ann Barnhart

Noncompliant* elderly persons are those individuals who, because of emotional, physical, or cognitive disabilities, pose severe problems and bewildering dilemmas for their caregivers. Whether in their own homes, the homes of family members, or institutional settings, elderly individuals struggle to maintain their dignity and independence. Ideally, caregivers—e.g., children, spouses, nurses, or aides—are dedicated to protecting the dignity and independence of those in their care. For the safety and well-being of the disabled elderly, caregivers sometimes find themselves in need of overriding the immediate wishes of those for whom they are responsible. It is, of course, important to understand that there are degrees of disability and degrees of intervention.[1]

---

*The term "noncompliance" is restricted to a therapeutic context in which elderly persons in the home or in institutional environments unreasonably resist or hinder the efforts of those working either to restore their physical and/or mental health or to make their lives more comfortable. Noncompliance must not be inflated to mean general noncooperativeness.

INSIDE INSTITUTIONS

Problem Areas

Noncompliant elderly patients create problems in at least four areas. First of all, they are problems to themselves, which is to say they often engage in behavior that comes into severe conflict with their own self-interest and with other activities that they wish to carry out. They become a problem to themselves because of dementia, physical illness, a decrease in functions, reduced capabilities, and loss of interests. Men in particular seem to dwindle if the job has been the dominant focus of their lives. "I am no longer a man" they say or think, as they sink into boredom and despair or increase their use of alcohol.

Carlyle entered the psychiatric treatment center after he had slept little, eaten little for a month, and had increased significantly his intake of alcohol. Now at the age of sixty-five, he has cirrhosis of the liver, a shrinking range of interests, and boredom as his constant companion.

Nellie's chronic pain, due in part to scoliosis* plus osteoarthritis, had gradually become the center and focus of her life. She had drawn up a long list of foods that she would not eat, and she refused to develop new activities or interests that promised to divert attention from her pain. It was as if suffering had become both her new identity and the magnet that attracted the social reinforcers she so desperately needed. Physicians were at her beck and call, and, like the Lady of the Manor, she required a special menu for herself. Staying in bed all of the time, she had learned that the bed was her throne from which she could rule those destined to serve her. In some respects, her illness was a mixed blessing, giving her power only so long as she remained in the thespian role of a suffering patient. A clever woman, she had in her own mind outwitted the nursing home staff. In other ways she had outsmarted herself in her confinement to the role of pain and misery.

Barbara, suffering from multi-infarct dementia,† must be constantly monitored in the special care unit. Fifteen minutes after being dressed, she will undress herself and slip back into the clothes that need to be laundered. If the staff fails to check on Barbara, she will wear the same clothing week after week. Having the normal desire for social interaction,

---

*Lateral curvature of the spine.

†Dementia associated with the combined effect of several small strokes or blockages of the blood supply in the brain.

she frustrates her own efforts by failing to recognize elementary social rules. For example, she moves uninvited into other patients' rooms or through the hallway to make intrusive conversation with staff, patients, or guests.

Because Helen did not work sufficiently hard in her physical therapy program, she must now, at the age of sixty-nine, live most of her waking hours in a wheelchair. Deeply frustrated and almost unbearably lonely, she yells out in the night and often during the day. When she wishes to eat, she yells for assistance. When she wishes to get out of bed, she yells. She yells when she must go to the bathroom. Very likely, yelling is more convenient for her than the simple act of pressing the call button. It is possible that she cannot process the world of technology. Yelling is only a minor problem to her but a major one to other patients and the staff. The staff becomes concerned when she shouts to the point of self-exhaustion. This, however, might be not so much a serious problem as a form of exercise for which she gets some attention but little praise.

In the second place, noncompliant elderly patients become problems not merely to themselves but to other patients.

Virginia, with advanced dementia, has been in a nursing home for two years, where she roams from room to room for the purpose of helping others and assuming a social role in the facility. Unfortunately her well-intended efforts are seldom helpful. Her help with the bathing and feeding of patients frequently turns into added work for the staff. She has become obsessive with one patient in particular, referring to the young woman as her granddaughter. Since the "granddaughter" is confined to a wheelchair, Virginia has "adopted" her and takes it upon herself to push the young woman down the halls despite the woman's protests. On one occasion Virginia pushed the patient through the double doors and outside the building. In addition, she insists on being present when the nurse bathes the younger woman. When staff members once tried to remove her from the scene, she became combative and inflicted an injury. Patients become combative with Virginia in their attempts to keep her out of their rooms.

Mabel's roommate reported that Mabel had hit her, whereupon Mabel was placed in a psychiatric center for evaluation and treatment. She was on a lowfat diet, but became angry and combative when she saw other patients being served bacon and eggs. On one occasion she hurled her tray across a dining room table. Mabel's life was not an easy one, for she had severe hearing impairment. When this was discovered, the staff began to understand her behavior. When she reacted to "insults," she very likely believed the comments directed to her were genuinely negative. Her hearing deficit, a possible stroke, and beginning dementia combined to turn a reasonably congenial and assertive woman into a defensive and assaultive patient who perceived her social world as intrusive, excessively free with unsolicited advice, and unaccepting of her. The world had become a threat to Mabel, and now she had become a threat to those around her. On one occasion she rushed up to a thirty-year-old man in a wheelchair and punched him in the face with her fist. She had misinterpreted his comment. On another day, Mabel became the recipient of a blow across the bridge of her nose. An equally hostile patient, thinking that Mabel had stolen her purse, removed her shoe and turned it into a weapon. After observing three incidents of shoes becoming weapons, the staff gave thought to proscribing hard-soled shoes.

In the third place, noncompliant elderly patients are problems to the staff. In fact, any conflict among patients can turn into a problem for the staff. For good reason, both patients and family members tend to hold the staff responsible when one patient injures another. The staff is expected to maintain law and order. Sometimes new staff members suffer role anxiety in the effort to sort out their multiple roles in the facility. Very often the roles are in conflict with one another. Staff members working closely with noncompliant patients can never forget that theirs is a job with some risk of violence.

Eighty-two-year-old Helton might appear to be a harmless old man, but he is in fact prone to violence. Standing six-foot-one, he is sexually aggressive. On one occasion he pinned a nurse to the shower wall, his huge hands gripping her like a vise. Four members of the staff were required to subdue him.

In the fourth place, noncompliant patients can create problems for their family members.

Sarah, age seventy-six and a diabetic, once had a phone in her room at the nursing home. When she became upset, she phoned family members long distance. At the end of the month the amount of her phone bill prompted her family to remove the telephone. The telephone can be a major line of abuse as well as communication between the patient and family members. It is often difficult to determine who creates problems —the patient or the family members. Noncompliant patients often possess the power to scuttle virtually any plan that the family members and the doctors may design to help them. Patients, however, sometimes perceive the family's plans as a means of taking control of their property and their lives.

The Question of Self-Determination

Granted that a "whole person" is something of a myth,[2] people who work with the difficult elderly come face to face with the disturbing question of the fragmenting self. As one family member said, "The Lord is taking my mother home piece by piece—on the installment plan." The thorny question of self-determination is made more complicated when the self seems to be riddled with lacunas. The problem of self-identity is difficult enough in the abstract, but with some of the elderly the mind seems to be a great jigsaw puzzle with major pieces missing. How can there be self-determination when the self is present only marginally? We do not like to think that the self exists in patches and degrees. We like to think of it as a complete unity. But those who work with the difficult elderly are reminded of the precariousness of the unity. It is disturbing to realize that in some cases the elderly person engaging in self-determination is not clearly the same self from day to day. The question "Who is in control?" keeps emerging.

As professionals we speak somewhat glibly of the individual's achievement of independence. In reality, each individual is dependent upon thousands of contingencies at every moment. The real question, therefore, has to do with the sources on which one depends and those other sources from which one wishes to be free. To be is to be related. To be is to be dependent. The confusion that is said to plague the elderly emerges largely because of the radical *rearrangement of sources of dependency* that shape their lives. Much of self-identity has to do with the sources and values *with* which one identifies. When there is a scrambling of sources and values, the elderly understandably suffer severe self-identity problems. This becomes intensified when one section of the brain ceases to be a reinforcing support to the rest of the brain and to the organism generally. The very concept of self-*interest* becomes problematic when the *self* cannot be easily identified.

THE NONCOMPLIANT ELDERLY AT HOME

Territorality is in the genes of virtually every species. Human beings are no exception, although as symbolic animals we have, for both good and ill, astounding flexibility in determining what shall be regarded as our territory. When the elderly continue to live in their own homes but need outside personal assistance, territorial conflict readily emerges. The helper coming into the home is always on the verge of being classified as an intruder. The truce is always on shaky ground.

Jane, an eighty-nine-year-old victim of Alzheimer's disease, knows that her kitchen is *her* kitchen. The stove is her territory. The helper must not invade that territory. So they have sandwiches for lunch. The bitter truth is that Jane cannot function at the gas stove and is in fact a danger to herself. The helper must always be alert to the odor of gas and be prepared to move quickly to prevent an explosion.

The elderly have had roles that, over the years, have defined their identity and their place in the world. When stripped of these roles, the victims either fight to recover them or fall into roles belonging to childhood or to other stages of life. In the home setting, because the territorial cues and the roles have been paired, considerable ambivalence and anger emerge when the link between territory and role is broken.

Jane's sixty-six-year-old daughter works downtown, but the phone makes her readily accessible. It is not uncommon for the daughter to receive calls of alarm from her mother. In most cases they are false alarms, but the responsibility of deciding what action to take in each case creates cumulative stress for the daughter.

When the brain begins to fail, it often does so without apparent design. Carolyn, age seventy, felt invaded by a woman she did not recognize. The intruder came into her home daily. In reality it was her own reflection in the mirror. Her brain had played a cruel trick on her.

LOOKING TO THE FUTURE

Briefly, those who care for the dependent elderly must come to terms with the invariably difficult and complicated question of self-determination when the self seems to exist as patches that are only loosely connected. The ethical question of respect for the self becomes acute and seemingly unmanageable when an individual seems to have little sustained pattern of self-interest.

All human social existence involves negotiation. In many cases the elderly lose their power or their right to participate in the process of negotiating their security and maintenance. Unfortunately, the assumption of responsibility presupposes the ability to respond to the cues essential for self-maintenance. When this ability begins to dissolve, the painful process of reevaluating the individual's responsibility for himself or herself emerges with a vengeance. It is very likely that the elderly, including the noncompliant, will need to have their right of counter-controls more practically defined. In many cases, they will need an advocate of some kind (not necessarily an attorney) to supplement their own loss of capacity to respond to the cues of self-interest.

There are certain avenues we must take as a humane society in order to meet the burgeoning financial, medical, and emotional problems of an aging population.

1. It is imperative that we set up more gerontological assessment centers for making comprehensive evaluations of elderly patients for earlier detection of problems. For example, we are now learning about the complex problems in medication use by the elderly.[3]

2. Professionals trained in behavior therapy are greatly needed in handling such problems as inappropriate toileting, yelling, hoarding, and acts of verbal and physical aggression.[4] The Omnibus Budget Reconciliation Act implemented in October of 1990 provides improved guidelines in managing chemical and physical restraints in long-term care facilities, and there is great challenge for creative care plans with alternate kinds of management.[5]

3. Eighty percent of the caregiving of the difficult elderly is done by family members. Whether it be providing hands-on care to a frail and dependent parent, making daily visits to prepare meals and give medications, or making numerous inquiries to find just the right services, the emotional and physical drain is enormous. Programs of respite care and assistance must be developed in every community.

NOTES

1. Some caregivers overstep their bounds in managing the difficult elderly. However, issues of mistreatment and abuse will not be covered in this paper.

2. Mary Ann and Joseph E. Barnhart, "The Myth of the Complete Person," in Mary Vetterling-Braggin, Frederick Elliston, and Jane English (eds.), *Feminism and Philosophy* (Towota, N.J.: Littlefield, Adams and Co., 1977), pp. 277–290.

3. Stephen C. Montamat, Barry J. Cusack, and Robert E. Vestal, "Management of Drug Therapy in the Elderly," *The New England Journal of Medicine,* 321, no. 5 (August 3, 1989):303–309.

4. Richard A. Hussian and Ronald L. Davis, *Responsive Care: Behavioral Interventions With Elderly Persons,* (Champaign, Ill.: Research Press, 1985).

5. Janice L. Feinberg, "Nonpharmacologic Alternatives to Chemical Restraints," *The Consultant Pharmacist,* 5, no. 7 (July 1990):370–388.

9

Long-Term Care:
The Women's Issue of the 1990s

Eva Skinner

Mary Taylor never thought it would end like this. An eighty-five-year-old widow, she is living her last years in a nursing home. Alone. Her sole income is Social Security, supplemented by the small savings she and her husband accumulated.

As a homemaker who occasionally worked part-time, she has no pension. The nursing home costs about twenty-five thousand dollars a year and Mary's money is fast disappearing since she must pay the charges herself. Soon she will have to turn to Medicaid to cover the nursing home costs. A woman whose pride in never having accepted a handout in her life is crushed as she helplessly spends down to impoverishment.

Before entering the nursing home, Mary lived alone and was cared for by her daughter and granddaughter, who lived nearby. They were unable to continue to care for her because of work, family responsibilities, and Mary's deteriorating health. Medicare would not pick up the cost of home health agency services—for which she had a limited amount of money. She was forced to enter a nursing home.

Mary has come face to face with *the* most frightening realization of older persons: the question "Who will take care of *me*?"

Mary's situation is hardly unusual. It illustrates, however, that long-term care is primarily a *women's* issue. After all, women are almost always both the primary receivers *and* providers of long-term care. Three out of four residents in nursing homes are women. The most likely candidate is a woman over eighty who—like Mary—lives alone.

Because of differences in longevity, older women are much more likely to be widowed than older men and, therefore, at greater risk of institutionalization. Two-thirds of all adults over age eighty-five are women. One out of every four women over eighty-five lives in a nursing home, with an even greater number needing help at home with personal care and homemaker services. Older women living at home have more functional limitations than older men. Only 28 percent of functionally impaired older women live with a spouse, compared with 73 percent of functionally impaired older men.[1]

Yet despite the fact that one out of two older Americans will spend some time in a nursing home during their lives, the great majority—over 70 percent—of those needing long-term care live in the *community* rather than in institutions.

Until recently, most people associated long-term care strictly with nursing home care. But the largest percentage of care is actually rendered in the home—by the family.

Approximately two-and-a-half million older Americans living in the community have difficulty performing personal care activities, such as getting dressed, bathing, walking, and preparing meals. They even have difficulty taking medication. These people need a combination of health care and social services to maintain their state of health and prevent deterioration. Maintenance depends on a *continuum* of care: doctor visits, home health care, adult day care, and—when necessary—nursing home care.

When one is elderly, *any* illness is more complex than for a young person: more complex emotionally and physically, not to mention economically—especially for women. Older women are more likely to have low incomes and often live at or below the poverty level. Needed care may be difficult to obtain—let alone afford.

In 1987, the last year for which government statistics are available, median income for women aged sixty-five and over was $6,734—57 percent of older men's median income. Only one out of five women over sixty-five receive income from pensions, either their own or their husbands'.[2]

One-third of all elderly unmarried women depend on Social Security for at least 90 percent of their income. The average monthly benefit for these women is a paltry $420. Yet these statistics tell only half of the story. Women traditionally have been considered society's nurturers and have taken on the role of caregiver in both their personal and professional lives. When care is needed for family members, the job invariably falls to the woman.

Of the nearly five million disabled persons living in the community, more than 70 percent rely exclusively on unpaid care provided by family and friends. Seventy-five percent of these caregivers are women—usually wives and adult daughters. According to a recent survey conducted by the American Association of Retired Persons, most caregivers provide care seven days a week—sometimes only a few hours each day, but *every* day.[3]

Age is no barrier to the demands of caregiving. The average age of women providing care to disabled spouses is sixty-nine; to disabled parents, fifty-two. Nearly half of these women describe their *own* health as fair to poor and nearly a third live in or near poverty. For these adult daughters, providing care for a very old and very sick parent can be literally overwhelming.

Then, of course, there is the "sandwich generation"—women with responsibilities for care of both children and parents at the same time. These caregivers—again usually adult daughters—must constantly balance multiple, competing demands. More than half are employed in the work force—one-out-of-two full-time. Those with children under age eighteen at home also number one-half.

Recent corporate studies show 20 to 30 percent of all full-time employees are caring for an elderly parent or other relative and significant numbers have been forced to scale back work hours—and thus their own standard of living—because of caregiving responsibilities. For them, the "36 hour day" is the norm rather than the exception.

Simply put, America's current long-term care policy—a policy where families, and thus women, are left to fend for themselves—is a tragic example of public policy gone wrong. It is both morally and ethically bankrupt.

We must make it right by developing a comprehensive long-term care system that meets the needs of functionally dependent persons of *any* age. To do so, the following objectives are paramount:

- Reform of the system must be comprehensive rather than incremental. It is not enough simply to tamper with one small part of the long-term care problem. A comprehensive approach is needed in which the entire scope of chronic illness is addressed—from acute hospitalization to the highest level of recovery possible.

- The system must correspond to the needs and preferences of functionally dependent persons and their families—correcting the current imbalance between institutional care and home- and community-based services.

- Eligibility for in-home and community long-term care services should be based on functional impairments and the need for assistance rather than on eligibility for institutional care.

- Individuals and their families must be provided the information they need to plan for possible financial, personal, and health-care crises should they become disabled or incapacitated. As well, they should understand—and be able to easily obtain—the legal tools they need to state their preferences about health-care treatments.

- There must be an effort to prevent the impoverishment of people who either require or deliver long-term care.

- The new system should be based on the principle of social insurance or "shared risk"—incorporating mechanisms designed to keep providers' costs at a reasonable level.

The system that is developed will very likely still require women to continue to provide the bulk of unpaid long-term care. Nonetheless, an equitable public policy—one that is truly humane—must recognize and provide supportive services to help facilitate this informal provision of care so that they and their families are not unreasonably burdened.

Let us not forget: there *have* been occasions during the last fifty years when our nation has had the political will and social conscience to adopt major legislation that helped aging families avoid economic catastrophe. In 1935, we created Social Security. Thirty years later, in 1965, we enacted Medicare. Now we realize that even together these two noble programs simply are not enough. The ruinous cost of long-term care—both economic and emotional—is *today's* catastrophe for aging families. For women in particular, it is truly a specter to be feared.

NOTES

1. Special Committee on Aging, *Developments in Aging: 1990*. Vol. 1, United States Senate, 1991.

2. Ibid.

3. Maryanne P. Keenan, *Changing Needs in Long-Term Care: A Chartbook* (Washington, D.C.: American Association of Retired Persons, 1989).

10

Lobbying Government for Long-Term Care

Ted Ball

The existing system of long-term care for the elderly in Canada is about
to undergo the most significant structural and program change since the
introduction of Medicare. Over the past couple of years, provincial governments from coast to coast have been conducting special commissions
of enquiry into their respective health and social-service systems. Many
have now established ongoing councils of health strategy—often reporting directly to the premier of the province—to plan how they should reform their long-term care, health, and social-service systems. There have
been major studies in the past two or three years on how to reform our
human service systems in virtually every province. And every one of these
enquiries has stated that unless we fundamentally restructure our health
and social-service systems, the nation will go bankrupt. The fact is that
we have developed a health-care system in Canada that is almost exclusively oriented to high-tech, high-cost institutions. We are one of the most
institution-crazy nations on earth. We actually institutionalize almost ten
percent of everybody over age sixty-five in Canada. We institutionalize
our elderly at almost twice the rate of any other industrialized nation on
earth.

Demographers and health-care economists have been warning us for
years that Canada is going to have to face a rapidly growing demand
for health and social services for the elderly in the 1990s. In 1986, 2.7

131

million Canadians were over sixty-five, representing 11 percent of the population compared to only 6 percent in 1931. By the year 2021, the percentage of seniors will increase to 19 percent when one out of every five Canadians will be a "senior." Since virtually 40 percent of all expenditures in our provincial health-care systems are for the elderly today, one can see why little beads of perspiration appear on the brows of provincial treasurers whenever anyone talks to them about the long-term health-care system in their province. They are increasingly convinced that if we were to maintain our existing structures and systems of care for the elderly, we would literally crush the taxpayers of this country.

Even before the real demographic boom takes place, we are already experiencing annual growth rates in provincial health-care spending that range between 10 and 12 percent annually across Canada. That is more than double the rate of inflation. But those growth rates are kid's stuff when one considers the cost pressures that will be brought about as our society continues to age over the next decade.

PRESSURES FOR REFORM

The fact is that we have to make some serious choices in this country if we want to maintain excellence within our long-term care system: we could double our current taxation rates; have everyone work an extra two days per week to increase our productivity as a nation; or fundamentally restructure our existing systems so that they are more efficient and cost-effective. What must be understood is that this is a very high-stakes game. Canada already has one of the highest per capita debts in the world. And the fact of the matter is that we are in serious economic trouble as a nation. We are paying almost forty billion (Canadian) dollars a year on just the interest charges on our national debt. That's the equivalent of the entire budget of the Province of Ontario.

It is important that providers of care for the elderly understand the pressures that are coming at them to change the way they do things and how they are organized. Provincial governments will be under extreme pressure over the next few years as a result of Ottawa's decision to address our national economic dilemma by reducing transfer payments to provinces. The harsh reality is that our national economy is carrying an accumulated debt load—much of it incurred from years of steady annual growth in spending under the Established Programs Financing Act (EPF) that pays the federal share of health care—which we cannot afford. Last year, EPF transfers to the provinces topped twenty billion dollars.

The reality is that from here on in, transfer payments to the provinces will decline in real terms. In fact, if provincial governments are not prepared to bite the bullet and reform their human-services systems, they will have to pay the additional costs through increased provincial taxes. That is why provinces are today scrambling to reform their existing systems of care for the elderly. And that is why each and every one of our programs is facing a "crisis" right now.

DANGERS AND OPPORTUNITIES

In Chinese the word "crisis" is represented by two word symbols: the symbol for "danger" and the symbol for "opportunity." Frankly, that is one of the best definitions of "crisis" I think anyone could devise, because the fact is that the long-term care system is faced with both danger and opportunity as it meets the reform challenges of the 1990s.

The purpose of lobbying to improve our system of care for the elderly is to maximize the opportunities and reduce the dangers. That will not be an easy task. The long-term care service sector is itself fragmented, competitive, and still fairly disorganized. Consumers at this point are, for the most part, weak and inarticulate about what they want. Nevertheless, service providers, consumers, and governments have common goals and objectives: all want an excellent yet affordable system of care for the elderly.

The opportunity that health-care professionals have is that by working together they could create a high-quality system of care that is co-ordinated, cost-efficient, and effective. But it is critically important that providers of care take a lead role in designing the new system that will be required in the 1990s. The danger is that if they are not prepared to actively help design the emerging system, they could be faced with bureaucratically imposed reforms that could lead to a down-grading of quality in the current system. Civil servants are under enormous pressure to put in place new delivery systems that are cost-efficient and well-managed. Caregivers have to work *with* them to ensure that a high level of quality and effectiveness in the system is maintained. Providers of care are now certainly under the gun. If they don't get their act together, then externally imposed reforms will simply wash over them. On the other hand, if they are prepared to be on the leading edge of reform as partners with government, the Canadians might just get the kind of care system for the elderly that seniors want and deserve.

Governments need and want the real-world knowledge health-care experts who can tell them how to improve the system. All caregivers should get actively involved in designing the new system in partnership with all levels of government.

CHALLENGES AHEAD

Let me make some blunt comments on the challenges that are ahead as provincial governments move toward the implementation of long-term care reform. First, we have to address the fact that we *are* overinstitutionalized. From here on in, we simply have to expand our community-based services for the elderly. Within the long-term care system, future growth has got to be concentrated on services that enable seniors to remain in their homes as long as possible, with their independence and dignity intact. Home-care programs, visiting nursing services, home-support programs, meals-on-wheels, and friendly visiting have to be key areas in which we concentrate growth in the future.

Second, remember that more than 80 percent of the care of elderly persons in this country is accomplished in an informal way by family caregivers. Public policy must shift to support those families—with expanded in-home services, respite care, counselling, financial support, and even tax incentives to assist families who agree to shoulder responsibility for their family members.

Third, the existing blur between "health" and "social services" must be addressed. In most provinces, there are still horrendous "gaps" in services for seniors in the health and social-services fields. And there is clearly a lack of coordination in the delivery of those programs. That has to change.

Demographers tell us that we are about to experience a 138 percent increase in the number of people over age eighty-five. These will primarily be women whose spouses have died. Prior to their inevitable decline in health status, their primary affliction will be loneliness. So, if we don't find creative ways to deal with that social affliction, these people will be heading for one of our already over-burdened institutions.

The challenge to long-term-care-system experts is to find ways to strengthen the front line of attack—the community-based, in-home service system and the kind of support that our institutions can give to family caregivers with services such as respite care and emergency relief. That should not diminish the role of institutional caregivers. It will simply slow the rate of demand for such services by shifting the system toward community-based care and slowing down the flow of patients to such facilities.

INSTITUTIONAL CARE

Most governments have decided basically that they won't build any new chronic care beds in the foreseeable future. But no one really knows what our needs for chronic and extended care beds will be in the middle or late 1990s. The reality of our demographics would indicate that we will need more beds in the future. Health-care professionals should be working with government to conduct independent assessments of bed requirements in the 1990s, assessments that take into account the projected impact of an expanded community-based system.

Collectively our society must reach decisions, based on realistic projections, about the need for capital growth in the long-term care system. Otherwise, we could have a crisis on our hands in a few years' time. There are also a number of other dangers faced by our institutional care providers in some of the "reforms" that are being projected for the 1990s. While there has been a strong lobby during the past decade to strengthen community-based care, governments may now be jumping on that bandwagon at the expense of institutional care. This is both dangerous and wrong.

Here in Canada, we have built one of the world's finest systems of institutional care for the elderly. Our nursing homes, homes for the aged, charitable homes, and chronic care hospitals are the backbone of our system of geriatric care. We have developed a genuine expertise and high levels of excellence in treating chronic disabilities. Our existing rehabilitation programs work miracles by regularly putting people back into the community as active, independent individuals who, with some home support, are able to lead active, productive lives. No one needs to apologize for coming from the institutional sector, he or she should be proud of it. Institutions play an incredibly valuable role in our society. The danger lies, however, in the government's newly found need to expand community-based care. This need could, quite possibly, allow our institutions to drift or deteriorate. That would be a tragedy and it should not be allowed to happen.

As our society progressively ages and the complexity of illness increases, our institutions will require further enrichment in staff if we are to maintain quality of care. So, as we move to create stronger linkages between our health and social-service systems, we have to ensure that we do not downgrade the quality of care in the existing system by deprofessionalizing it. In fact, we presently have a shortage of physiotherapists, speech-language pathologists, audiologists, and occupational therapists. If our society is going to meet the challenge of the 1990s, we had better begin producing more of these professionals.

Providers of care should work closely with government to ensure that investment continues to expand in rehabilitation and activation programs in aggressive treatment and chronic care hospitals as well as in nursing homes and homes for the aged.

MINIMUM STANDARDS

Another strategy that most provinces are considering is the decentralization of the decision-making system within long-term care, as well as within health and social-service systems. District health councils, or local planning authorities reporting to community boards and local provincial civil servants will be making decisions on everything from what services should be offered to the rate of payment for services. But without a comprehensive set of *standards* for levels of care services, and without an agreed upon set of *core programs* that should be available in each community, local planning authorities could end up doing whatever they want. Caregivers should be working with the government and consumers to develop those minimum standards. Most provinces are now moving toward the single-access agency model* that has been pioneered in Alberta. While the concept makes a great deal of sense, consumers and providers of care should maintain vigilance to ensure that "consumer choice" remains supreme. We have to ensure that an appropriate balance is struck between the maximum efficiency of the system and the individual preferences of the consumers. If we develop autocratic facility placement systems, consumers will revolt. It is as simple as that: access to the system has to be logical and fair, but it must also be sensitive to consumer preferences.

Providers of care should also lobby governments for improved salaries, continuing education programs, and increased administrative support. If home-care services are indeed to be in the front line of reformed long-term care, they need to be strengthened immediately. Existing low wages and higher turnover rates in staff at both the provider and administrative levels simply must be addressed. If home-care organizations are going to expand rapidly over the next few years, then it would be prudent if government would significantly increase funding to support the development of enhanced administrative, financial, and planning skills within existing management structures. Providers of care should, therefore, be lobbying for continuing education programs and increased administrative support.

CONSUMERS

When the long-term care sector approaches government, it would be well advised to have the support of consumer groups. In fact, consumers should

---

*Single access model refers to the case management of an individual by a single agency responsible for determining access to the long-term care facility most appropriate for the person's need (i.e., nursing home, residential facility, etc.)

be involved at every level of policy-advocacy development, for consumers and providers are allies in the debate about long-term care reform. Professional caregivers should work with them through coalitions and joint submissions to government.

WORKING TOGETHER

First, professionals and nonprofessionals alike must begin to work together as a sector. Chronic-care hospitals, nursing homes, home-care agencies and the professions involved in caring for the elderly should meet and plan together regularly.

When federal and provincial governments claim that the long-term care sector is fragmented and disorganized, they are right. This sector doesn't have any real history of working cooperatively. Traditionally, there has only been sporadic contact between providers of care. But caregivers must approach government with coherent and constructive advice from the entire long-term care sector. Quite frankly, there should be greater cooperation and coordination between the for-profit and the not-for-profit sectors involved in long-term care. Both are going to grow, and they have more in common than they have differences; therefore, they should work together.

We must understand that governments are scrambling to put in place a system of care for the elderly that will meet the demands of the 1990s in a cost-effective way. The task of health-care providers is to become active partners in the design of new approaches.

REFORM IN ONTARIO

The government of Ontario has just released the most comprehensive strategy for long-term care produced anywhere. "Strategies for Change," as it is called, is a most comprehensive articulation of where government thinking in Canada is headed. The strategy is to rapidly expand community-based care and to introduce an entirely new approach to decentralized decision making in the allocation of resources within the system.

At first glance, Ontario's strategy appears to have a somewhat anti-institutional and anti-professional bias. That might reflect the desire to force the pendulum to swing in the direction of community-based care, but it could also downgrade our institutions if we fail to maintain an appropriate balance within the system. I am not convinced that government fully appreciates the value of the role of rehabilitation, or the role that our institutions play in returning frail elderly people back into the community. The reality is that elderly people get sick, get treatment, and return to their homes. The role of the chronic-care hospital, and the many nursing homes that have advanced rehabilitation programs, is critically important to our long-term care system.

It may be appropriate for the pendulum to swing toward the community-based sector, but it is important to ensure that, as it does, the excellent network of long-term care facilities is not neglected. That is why the long-term care sector must work with government to develop policies, programs, and funding mechanisms that recognize the need to expand community-based services while ensuring the continual enhancement of the capabilities of our institutional sector.

LOBBYING GOVERNMENT

As a consultant specializing in public-affairs management, I can tell you what I think will be the ingredients of a successful lobby for long-term care reform. The success of such a lobby will depend on:

1. *The extent to which the argument is focused on the "public interest"*: Arguing for *standards* of care and *core programs* of service with the active support of consumers will be effective. As we move toward the devolvement of our system to the local level, we must be certain that citizens are guaranteed a minimum level of available services. That's a "public interest" argument, and everyone should be working together as a sector to make such arguments with the support of consumers.

2. *The extent to which there is consensus within the long-term care sector in specific provinces*: If all components of the long-term care sector work together instead of competing with each other, they will constitute a far more powerful force when dealing with government. Traditionally, there has been a high degree of mistrust and competitiveness between the component parts of the long-term care system, which, unfortunately, reinforces the government's view of that sector as fragmented and cantankerous. Working together allows for strength in unity.

3. *The extent to which health-care groups are organized to communicate with both governments and the grassroots of their organizations*: When going to the government such organizations must have their act together in terms of policy assessment and analytical skills. Their challenge is to work in partnership with government decision makers and planners so that a balance is struck between expertise and real-world

knowledge of the system with government's skills in policy and program development. By working together the collaboration will create a system that maintains quality at an affordable price to the taxpayer. But all health care groups must be sure that they have the complete support of the grassroots of their organizations and have involved them in the development process of the organizations' advocacy positions. For provincial organizations, this is critical, for as we move to local decision-making authorities, the strength of provincial organizations will depend on the strength of their individual agencies. In fact, if provinces do decentralize to the local level decisions on the allocation of resources, then it will be the local agencies, branches, and facilities that will have to negotiate their rates of pay or global budget with the local authority. So, programs must be developed that devolve government relations and government negotiating skills down to the local level.

4. *The extent to which a position is sold to members of provincial legislatures, bureaucrats, ministers, and the media:* This requires organization and the development of the same calibre of organized lobbies as that of hospitals and physicians in any province, otherwise health-care providers will not be serious players in the determination of reforms for the long-term care system.

Once positions have been developed, communicate them to all of the decision makers at the bureaucratic and political levels and use the media to reach consumers. This does not mean going to war with the government; it means ensuring that the debate on options and approaches is being conducted in full view of the public. From my personal experience of working in Ontario, I can say that I have never seen a more dedicated and hard-working group of health-care organizations and agencies.

We know that governments should build an affordable high-quality system for long-term care in this country. We have the experts. If they can work together as charitable homes, nursing homes, homes for the aged, chronic-care hospitals, visiting homemakers and nurses, volunteer groups and consumers, they will be a most powerful voice. And by working in partnership with government, they will accomplish improved co-ordination within the long-term care sector.

I am convinced that if caregivers are prepared to organize, to work together with consumer groups, to work as a sector and invest their time and energy on lobbying for high-quality care of the elderly, they will succeed in developing a high-quality, cost-effective long-term care system that will meet the needs of the 1990s and beyond. The future of long-term care is truly in their capable hands.

11

The Role of the Geriatrician

Peter N. McCracken

What do I believe is the role of the geriatrician in the 1990s? The questions we ought to pose right at the beginning are:

Who is the geriatrician and what does he or she do?

Who is the carer of the elderly, and is this carer synonymous with the geriatrician?

Although some of my colleagues might present a different definition, to me the role of the geriatrician is to function as a clinician, as an educator, as a researcher, as a role model, and as a health-care planner.

THE GERIATRICIAN AS A CLINICIAN

When I came to Alberta in 1988, there was only one certified geriatrician ahead of me. While it was important for me to initiate dialogues, go to meetings, and do planning, it was also important for the health-care planners and for the people in administration to notice that I saw patients. So I put on my white coat every day and spent a number of hours making rounds and seeing patients. I think this activity of the geriatrician is very important.

The buzz word in health care, particularly in university settings, is "assessment," geriatric assessment. The purpose of geriatric assessment is to enable old people to maintain optimum health, fitness, and independence and to ensure that they retain maximum control over their lifestyle with the same range of choice as the other adults in their society. The plan of action for the geriatrician, besides assessment, is to initiate treatment, to bring in rehabilitation, to effect primary care, and to ensure case coordination and appropriate use of resources.

There are four components to the geriatric patient.

1. *Age changes.*
   Aging isn't static and predictable; it's dynamic. Different organs within the same body age at different times. Different people of the same race age at different speeds. A person can have a set of thirty-year-old lungs and a fifty-year-old heart. A vague rule of thumb is that there is a one percent loss of reserve in our systems every year after age thirty.

2. *Age acquired illnesses.*
   Often once an illness is diagnosed, that diagnosis stays with the patient forever. Arthritis, osteoporosis, peripheral vascular disease, stroke, emphysema, diabetes, and so on, are like rocks in a knapsack that the elderly carry with them from that point on.

3. *Psychosocial precariousness.*
   Older patients are isolated, their friends die, their children move out of town, and they are left alone. Their supports in the community often evaporate.

4. *Tendency toward illness.*
   The elderly are the subset in our population more prone to acute illness—e.g., new pneumonias, new infections, heart failure—than any other segment of our population. Old people need good physicians, professionals who will put their fingers into the armpit and really examine lymph nodes, listen carefully to hearts and lungs, watch how elders walk, and assess them carefully.

Geriatric assessment has four parts: a physical workup, a mental status assessment, an assessment of functional aspects, and an assessment of social supports. Leave out any one of the four and the assessment is incomplete. The geriatric team includes the physician, the nurse, the physical therapist, the occupational therapist, the social worker, and perhaps other health professionals such as a psychologist, a pharmacist, a recreational therapist, a chaplain, a speech therapist, and a chiropodist. Without the team, geriatric medicine cannot function fully. Diagnosing old people is compounded by the fact that their disease may appear differently than in the young and the middle-aged. Elder physiology is different; elders have much less reserve. They often have several conditions ongoing simultaneously with a mixture of new and old diseases wrapped up in one person. They often have too many medications. In 1984, California geriatrician Larry Rubenstein conducted a controlled double-blind study. His two-year follow-up showed that geriatric assessment resulted in improved functional status on discharge, lowered mortality rates, reduced medication usage, improved mental status, increased return to the community, and fewer acute nursing home days. Geriatric assessment works.

Who should get a geriatric assessment? Basically and ideally the patients with confused states; those susceptible to falls; those presenting problems with mobility; any who experience incontinence, psychosocial breakdown, new acute medical and surgical illness; those with foreseeable difficulties in discharge; and all who seek institutional placement.

Geriatric assessment must include awareness of the multiple problems that people have. When I went to medical school, I was taught to unite all the factors in the history and all the findings on the physical exam into a single diagnosis. How things have changed! Most of my patients have five, six, or seven problems going on at the same time, all feeding in and interrelating, so the single diagnosis approach to disease is inadequate for geriatrics. In addition, old people tend to under-report their problems. The popular concept is that they over-report, but that's just not so. Doctors take blood pressure, look in the throat, listen to the heart and lungs, tap on the reflexes, probably give a prescription, and dismiss the patient. With old people the focus has to be widened. Consider the medication effect, check vision and hearing, look at the mouth and the teeth, look into bowel and bladder functions, examine the feet, look at mobility, ask about falls, and check on sleep patterns. These are the elements of the widened medical focus.

The requisites for adequate geriatric assessment include:

1. *Time.*

   It's tough to do a geriatric assessment in an emergency room, but if time is limited to twenty minutes, it is not possible to do an adequate assessment.

2. *Space, a table, and help.*

   A geriatrician can spend fourteen and a half minutes just taking off the seven layers of clothing that an elderly patient may wear.

3. *A complete detailed history.*

This history should include present and past problems as well as psychiatric problems and a history of their social situation. With a ninety-year-old the question "Do you have any chest pain?" is no more important than "Are you living by yourself or are you living with somebody?" The medical focus has to change.

4. *Assessment of social resources including relatives and friends.*

Many elderly people cannot give a clear history. It becomes important to use the telephone to check on how a patient is feeling two weeks, four weeks, and six weeks before he or she is admitted to the emergency room. This important information often seems to be omitted.

5. *A complete medical assessment.*

Of particular importance are the neurological examination, the postural blood pressure, and not a single blood pressure but two. Take a blood pressure with the patient lying flat, then stand the patient up and take a second blood pressure. If possible have the patient walk around for a couple of minutes, then take a third blood pressure. You'd be surprised how many people have what we call orthostatic hypotension, their blood pressure falls when they stand up. Sometimes it's symptomatic, sometimes it isn't. If you're going to prescribe medication for elderly patients, you should know if they have orthostatic hypotension. Check hearing and vision, do a rectal examination, look at mobility. The "get up and go" test—where the patient gets up, walks a short distance, and then sits down in a chair—can provide important information about function. Doctors coming out of medical school aren't taught to focus on an elderly person's gait.

6. *Construct a medical problem list.*

That's simple enough. Make sure the list is complete, then go on to functional assessment. Those who work in nursing homes understand the importance of bathing, dressing, toileting, walking, feeding, and transfers. These are the basic domestic activities of daily living. Often a physician just does the screening part and it is the occupational therapist who delves in and gets the valid information. Instrumental activities of daily living include housekeeping, cooking, shopping, banking, paying bills, and travel. Can the elder handle all of these responsibilities? If not, then obviously these needs are going to have to be addressed when doing discharge planning.

7. *Make a functional problem list.*

The key to this is to try to make it as complete as possible without rushing the job.

8. *Match the medical and functional problem lists.*

Identify a disability gap that occurs when the medical problems don't explain the functional problems. When a medical problem list doesn't add up to a functional problem list, only a few possibilities remain. Either the medical problem list is inaccurate, the functional problem list is inaccurate, or there's a disability gap.

9. *List all the medication the patient is taking.*

If there isn't a medical reason for the medication, discard it. So many older people take medications they don't absolutely need. Sometimes it's the physician's fault, sometimes it's the patient's fault. Some patients visit several doctors and stockpile pills that aren't needed.

10. *Design appropriate investigative steps.*

This includes treatment, assessment, rehabilitation, and discharge planning.

Geriatric assessment requires flexibility. Not every person over sixty-five requires such an assessment. The setting of an assessment can be a geriatric facility, a long-term care setting, or the home, and it can be done by community nurses who can consult with geriatricians if there are specific medical problems. Assessment-targeting will be important in the 1990s. Some provinces have a relatively limited geriatric assessment unit requiring selection of what people should be assessed. This means that a lot of people are going to be left out, which reflects the situation existing before geriatric medicine came along. I work in a facility where there are 180 geriatric assessment beds so the issue of targeting doesn't really confront me. My colleagues and I take seriously ill patients and hope to get them up and moving. In other provinces, in other settings, when the geriatric assessment unit has only ten or twelve beds, physicians have to be selective of patients.

About fifteen to twenty years ago, confused patients in the hospital were not addressed at all. Now, the pendulum has swung: when a patient becomes confused there's a tendency to label them as having Alzheimer's disease. Remember, confusion is a symptom just as chest pain is a symptom. Elderly people can become confused because they are medically sick, because of medication, or because they are depressed. Patients should be completely assessed before labels like Alzheimer's disease or dementia are attached. The demented patient with behavioral disturbance presents a special problem in long-term care centers. Agitation, apathy, sleep disturbances, paranoid ideation, hallucinations, and, finally, agitation and violence create problems for which there are no adequate coping responses.

Geriatric education of physicians, health-care workers, nurses, rehabilitation workers, social workers, and so on, is primary to prevent medical ageism. This attitude, which usually develops in medical school or resident training, manifests itself by avoidance—emotional, intellectual, and physical—of elderly patients, and leads to pessimism about the outcome of therapeutic intervention. We know that old people do well with certain kinds of interventions and treatments and that they can bounce back. But medical ageism is blind to that fact. It implies that old people could not possibly have diseases worthy of discussion in medical schools or university hospitals. Fortunately this attitude is being changed. On the other side of medical ageism is doctor-bashing, which can only produce negative results within the long-term care sector. It is alleged that physicians don't spend enough time with old patients and that they get angry when the elderly try to talk to them. I submit that physicians don't do remarkably well when one considers how little training they receive in medical school about how to take care of older people. Few receive training in how to function as part of a team, unless they are recent graduates. So be patient with doctors. Give them credit for what they do.

Modern medical school geriatric education must include the theory and mechanism of aging, learning to distinguish normal from pathological aging, training in history-taking and the physical examination of older people, and development of appropriate communication and interpersonal skills. Education in geriatric assessment is paramount and includes information about how to assess someone who falls, how to properly handle the person with urinary incontinence, and how to try to improve patients to get them functioning on a higher level. Geriatricians need to know how to assess, diagnose, and manage dementia and how to talk with the family and set up the discharge possibilities to enable a patient to move back into the community.

This year one half of the fourth-year medical students at the University of Alberta will do a month of geriatric medicine. Every family-medicine resident will do a month of geriatric medicine. Our geriatric-medicine training program has four trainees in it now and will have four more next year.

THE GERIATRICIAN AS RESEARCHER

Obviously the importance of doing research cannot be overemphasized. Research in aging and health care of the elderly, like geriatric medicine itself, is in its infancy. If we are going to find answers to dementia, incontinence, osteoporosis, and many of the illnesses that beset the elderly, research must be a top priority. We are doing some research in urinary incontinence, which is the involuntary loss of urine of sufficient quantity or frequency to be a social health problem. Presently it is undertreated due to decreased reporting by patient's under-recognition, lack of education in this area, inadequate staffing in long-term care facilities, and gaps in medical sophistication. We cannot cure ischemic heart disease, diabetes, or osteoarthritis. We can only help patients achieve a higher level of comfort. In the case of urinary incontinence, we can't cure it but we can make it easier to manage thereby requiring less staffing, less linen, and so on. Research in urinary incontinence in the elderly and the neurogenic control of bladder function is underway.

THE GERIATRICIAN AS A ROLE MODEL

I think it's important for geriatricians to convey their interest in old people to students and other physicians in the field. If a geriatrician can't get excited about treating an elderly patient then who will? When it comes to being the role model, there's no substitute for wearing your heart on your sleeve as you function as a geriatrician.

In an institution, a geriatric role model is one who digs in and functions with pride and with as much independence as possible. The geriatric role model is someone who says send me what you've got and we'll give it everything we have. We may not cure the patient, the patient may die, but we're not going to push the eject button. If a patient becomes disturbed and difficult to handle, it is not necessary to push the eject button. The nursing staff, the recreational therapist, and the doctor can sit down and, with pride in the institution, try to care for the patient through this difficult period.

Presently, the tendency is to reject elderly problem patients and transfer them to another facility: from an acute care hospital to a convalescent hospital to the nursing home and then back again. The role model should not push the eject button.

THE GERIATRICIAN AS HEALTH-CARE PLANNER

In terms of health-care planning, a regional health-care program is the goal and the idea, because the regional plan guarantees, or tries to guarantee, that geriatric assessment goes on no matter where the patient happens to be. In reality, geriatric medicine and assessment is centered on acute-care hospitals. When the ninety-one-year-old lady breaks down, she doesn't go to a geriatric assessment facility or to a nursing home; she goes to the emergency room of a hospital, and that is where we need geriatric medicine and assessment. Any regional program will have to include the acute-care hospitals. Home care is also a vital component of a regional plan. People must be looked after and assessed and supported within their own homes. There can be no regional plan without a home-care component. As a health-care planner, a geriatrician tries to coordinate specialized facilities and acute-care hospitals.

I would like to conclude with a personal comment on the role of the geriatrician as a dreamer about the future. When I first arrived in Edmonton, at a beautiful facility of bricks and mortar with lots of human resources, I had this dream that some day there would be a program here, with medical students and nonphysicians in training at an academic facility that would develop geriatrics in conjunction with the acute-care hospitals in the city. As I visited patients I couldn't get the idea out of my mind and it is now beginning to evolve. I think as we talk about some of the choices for Canada in the 1990s, we need to remember that dreams can come true.

12

Geroethics

Gerald A. Larue

Any discussion of long-term care for the coming decade must include an appreciation of gerontological ethics or "geroethics," by which I mean the consideration of ethical, moral, and value issues as they pertain to elders. My focus will be primarily on those who today are sixty-five years of age and older, but it includes those who will become elders in the twenty-first century, the century that some have labeled "the retirement century." I propose to make some general statements pertaining to elder ethics and then touch on five specific issues. Finally, I will suggest a basic, guiding ethic for eldercare and elder life.

Today's elders are survivors. They have survived more dramatic changes in lifestyles, education, science, technology, communication, and internationalism than have ever before been made in one generation. They have survived devastating childhood diseases, wars, depression, and inflation. They are the doers who have brought the present into being, who have contributed to making the United States and Canada, and indeed the world, what they are today.

The primary ethical questions are: What do we owe these elders? What, if anything, have they earned through their long years of contribution to the growth, stability, and well-being of the nation? Can they claim any priority by virtue of age over other, younger citizens? Are there moral or ethical requirements to provide care for elders, care that equals or exceeds care for others? For example, does a child in a neonatal facility deserve medical care and treatment equal to or surpassing that of a frail elder hospitalized in an intensive care unit? In both instances, life is sustained by modern medical technology administered by a skilled staff and paid for out of public funds. Medical care given to the infant holds the promise of saving a potentially productive and useful life of many years. But does that fact make the infant's life more valuable and more deserving of care than that of an elder whose life trajectory is near completion? Should equal amounts of time and money be provided? How valuable, how important are elders?

Do we employ triage when deciding whom to treat—that principle which came into being during military emergencies when, because of scarcity of medicines, doctors, and nurses, injuries were prioritized and the wounded were treated, not on a first-come-first-served basis, but according to estimates of which injuries could be successfully treated and which showed little hope of survival? Do we decide that upon reaching a certain age, only limited care should be available to elders? Before examining the ethical implications of these questions, I will touch on some other basic concerns.

Principles influencing the treatment of elders in Western society are derived from Judeo-Christian traditions and Greek rationalism; they include concepts of beneficence and nonmaleficence. Beneficence stresses the importance of doing good for others and embraces the responsibility to prevent harm, to remove harmful conditions, and to provide positive benefits that cater to longer and better life, including relief from pain, suffering, and illness, and the enhancement of human functioning. Nonmaleficence calls for acts that do not harm others and stems from the belief in the sanctity of human life and the need to protect life.

The most feasible ethical philosophy for a nation is utilitarianism, which asserts that we ought to seek the greatest possible balance of value over disvalue, and which, in the name of utility, calls for policies that provide the greatest benefits for the greatest number. But, we live in a democracy that respects the principle of personal autonomy and freedom to choose, and honors the right of individuals to act on personally chosen plans. Without such personal autonomy, life becomes limited, contained, boxed in, and denied its full potential. The principle of autonomy protects personal integrity by denying others, even governmental trustees, the right to invade and dictate an individual's lifestyle or living patterns. Autonomy may be thwarted by social situations, living conditions, poverty, extreme illness, or mental deterioration. In such instances, the principle of benevolence calls for intervention by properly authorized personnel to act on behalf of and for the well-being of the individual elder. When intervention becomes the responsibility of the gov-

ernment, questions of cost and the distribution of national resources become relevant.

We are a decent and caring people. We recognize a moral responsibility to provide help to those in need. Our national ethic recognizes the
equal worth of all and calls for beneficent responses. We begin by agreeing
on a basic survival ethic that guarantees food, clothing, housing, security,
and protection of personal property to all thereby freeing citizens from
fear of abject poverty. But is this enough?

Life in this great nation has always been evaluated as something more
than mere existence. Quality of life calls for experiencing feelings of self-
fulfillment, self-actualization, personal worth, and self-control. Help
provided for elders should be designed to encourage independence and
personal responsibility.

If anything has become clear from research in aging, it is that individuals age differently and react differently to the aging process. The danger in utilitarianism applied to aging is the tendency to ignore the unique
life patterns of individual elders and focus on the greatest good for the
greatest number. Of course, no single approach can possibly satisfy every
elder, and any attempt to develop policy to meet every individual need
could result in chaos. What is called for, then, is not rule-book ethics,
but situation ethics; it recognizes that differing life situations call for different responses—even though they may not appear in the rule book.

Demographics provides us with relatively reliable estimates of the
number of elders who will reach sixty-five or seventy-five or eighty-five
years of age at any given time. We can calculate the number who are
likely to require long-term care. What the numbers cannot tell is how
individual elders will react to retirement, to entry into nursing care facilities, to reduction in income, to the realization that they have entered a
social discard heap where it it is tacitly assumed that they have little or
nothing to contribute to the present or future. Elders are men and women
who have enjoyed the freedom to make personal choices. With age, their
choices can become severely limited, and if those limitations are governed
by some need to conform to an established rule-book ethic enhanced by
utilitarian patterns, then their individuality will be ignored. It is far easier
for administrators to provide rules than it is for free-thinking elders to
have their specific life situations ignored and to be treated according to
"the book." The conflict between rule-book ethics and situational ethics
is basic. Now let's look at some ethical issues that relate to the problem.

The first ethical issue pertains to individualism. Each elder brings to
any environment a unique personal background reflecting what was experienced in life, how the experience was interpreted, and whether the
experience was helpful or damaging. Each brings personal biases,

prejudgments, dogmas, and distortions as well as qualities of spirit, coping, and temperament. For better or for worse, each elder affects the environment of which he or she is a part. Some are nourishing individuals whose ability to adjust, whose humor, openness, and wisdom make their presence a pleasure. Others, who are just the opposite, bring toxic influences into almost every setting. What we cannot know is what each elder carries in terms of inner conflicts never resolved, terrible damage that was never repaired, psychological wounds that were never treated. Without knowledge of the internal burdens, we cannot understand the elder. Let me illustrate.

Emily was sixty years old and had been married for forty-two years when she was widowed. After the funeral she went into a sudden decline. She could not walk and soon found herself in a wheelchair. She seemed unable to carry out the most ordinary of tasks. She became a helpless burden to everyone. Yet a thorough medical examination found no basis for her condition.

Then a social worker asked the right questions. This woman who had moved so graciously and confidently in social circles had never been permitted to mature or take care of herself. Emily was married right out of high school to a man already well along in his career and he had looked after her. She had never learned to drive a car; he had always arranged for her transportation. She had never learned to write checks or balance accounts; her husband had provided charge accounts at the various stores, and when plastic charge cards were invented she used those. He had always paid the bills. Emily was a helpless woman when the social worker took her in charge.

Today she drives her own car, handles her finances, and appears more poised and at ease than she ever was during her many years of marriage. No one knew the insecurity and feelings of helplessness and inadequacy that she carried inside. Without much information it was not possible to understand that her demanding, childlike dependency and her sudden physical helplessness were simply protective coverings.

When I met Harvey, he was sixty-eight years old and in a state of severe decline. After rising to a responsible position on the corporate ladder, he had retired at age sixty-five, in accordance with company policy. He had numerous friends and was a welcome guest in many homes. Harvey had been a widower since the age of fifty-five and had become quite a lady's man. After retirement he made bad investments and ultimately went bankrupt. He moved from a comfortable apartment in a better section of the city to a single room in a rather seedy neighborhood. He underwent a triple by-pass heart operation. Harvey felt that his life was falling apart. He refused all invitations from former friends because he felt he could not come to their door as he once had with a bottle of expensive wine under his arm, nor could he repay their invitations. He looked at his financial status and felt that he was a failure in their eyes, just as he was a failure in his own. He believed his former lady friends would reject him because he was impotent. He needed counseling but could not afford the best therapists, and he refused the services of free clinics. His world, his life, and his personality began to shrink. Why?

Harvey had grown up committed to the work ethic. In his mind, people were accepted on the basis of job status—what they earned, what they did, how well they succeeded. He could not believe that friends wanted him as a guest just because of who he was. Harvey could not accept being liked for himself, for his warm personality and his friendliness. And he could not accept the fact that women were drawn to him because they found in him qualities of gentleness, respect, and understanding, not because of his sexual performance. Harvey's doctor explained that his impotence was not due to physical problems, but rather because he suffered from low self-esteem and believed he was a failure and would fail at anything he attempted.

I saw him only once in an extended session, and then he dropped out of sight. He had carried into his retirement a work ethic that gave rise to notions, beliefs, and ideas about life and about himself that proved to be destructive and life-threatening. I was convinced that if he did not get counseling, the depression would deepen and ultimately bring on an early death.

Agnes was also retired. She was sixty-nine and suffered from a mylenization*of the spinal cord that produced pain and limited her mobility to the use of a walker. She lived in a comfortable two-bedroom house with her ninety-year-old husband. Agnes was an angry woman. She shouted at the day workers who were provided to help with household chores and meal preparation. They did "dumb things": they put the spoons on the right-hand side of the cutlery drawer rather than left, they replaced toilet paper rolls with the sheets hanging next to the wall rather than on the outside.

Agnes wanted to commit suicide. Why? Her pain was under control. She was being cared for. She had many years of life ahead. Her husband was a kind, gentle, and caring man. Why did she want to die?

Inside, Agnes carried responses to life that grew out of a destructive

---

*The disease or destruction of the fatlike substance surrounding groups of nerves, such as the spinal cord.

childhood. After her mother and father divorced, her mother entertained lovers, and Agnes, from age eight on, was molested by these men. She was placed in a foster home and was molested again. The second and third foster homes were no better, so she ran away at age thirteen. She found work and continued her education on her own until she graduated from high school. Then she met Leon, they married, and had a son who eventually became an engineer. Agnes was a fighter. She was independent. She and Leon supported social causes for the outcasts, the unfortunate, and underprivileged. She joined marches and picket lines. Now she and Leon lived a relatively comfortable retired life, and she wanted to die.

Agnes had fought to be independent. It was the only lifestyle she trusted. As a child she learned that when she was dependent on others, bad things happened to her. Now, with helpers to care for her house, to accompany her on her daily walk down the block, she felt dependent, and the damage experienced in childhood, long since buried, now surfaced in anger and resentment at her helplessness. Life under such circumstances was not worth living. Ultimately she took her own life by grinding up and swallowing a fatal mixture of medications. There were those who could understand neither her anger nor her suicidal intentions, because they did not know or understand what she had brought into her old age from childhood.

On the other hand, there are courageous, loving elders who cope with traumatic illness in ways that are moving testimonials to the power of love. Hortense, a trained social worker, married a brilliant businessman who contracted Alzheimer's disease. By age seventy he had declined mentally to a childlike state. One day he asked Hortense the same simple question over and over again, at least a dozen times. Each time she patiently answered. Finally she lost control and snapped at him. "At that moment," she recalled, "I looked at him and he stood there like a crestfallen child. Then he said, 'I only want you to love me, honey.' What could I do? I put my arms around him and held him. After all, he was still the man I loved, even though he was no longer the man I married."

Hortense had grown up in a loving, caring family. She brought to the marriage the loving, caring, supportive personality that had motivated her to choose a career in social work. When her husband's mind began to fail, that same nourishing, caring personality moved her to care for him until he died. Today she is an eighty-year-old dynamo, actively involved with Alzheimer's and gerontology programs and still in love with life.

Each elder is an individual, who carries the burdens, the failures, and the triumphs of the past. Some have raw emotional wounds that can still bleed and drain energy. Others have inner beauty that can transform any situation.

The ethical principle I am stressing can be simply phrased in the words of that famous Indian proverb, *"Do not judge another until you have walked a mile in his moccasins."*

The second ethical issue grows out of the first and is related to the fact that we have entered a no-deposit-no-return era. Whatever may be classified as used or worn out, out-of-date or nonfunctional should be replaced or discarded. There are those who would place the feeble elderly in this category. Elders are viewed as expensive commodities who do not contribute to social growth. They have served their purpose. They can be profitably replaced by younger men and women in the workplace. They should be put out to pasture, to use a farm analogy, or placed on a back shelf and forgotten. Some are put out to pasture and others do end up on back shelves, virtually forgotten. These are the frail or chronically ill who may be emotionally disturbed, abusive, cantankerous, or given to the use of drugs or alcohol. They may hallucinate or be unsure of where or who they are. They need help. What can be done with them? Who wants to look after them?

Some end up in board-and-care facilities so ill equipped to handle their individual needs, so understaffed, so unsanitary, that few would find the setting tolerable. They are left to the mercies of caregivers for whom the best interests of elders may not be a priority. No one hugs these outcasts, no one touches them except, perhaps, in a professional bedside manner. As human discards, they have become our untouchables and made to feel that they do not really matter to anyone. There is toxic potential in such treatment.

Studies have demonstrated that the need for touch is basic to human health. James Prescott has argued, on the basis of his research, that lack of touching in infancy is a precursor to violence. When elders are subtly placed in the untouchable category, when caregivers make only minimal physical contact with them, they know they have been discarded. Some feel they have become so unattractive that others hesitate to touch them.

Only recently have our medical schools started to emphasize the importance of appropriate touching of elders. Helen Colton, in her book *The Gift of Touch,* has published a personal letter from Dr. Stephen R. Smith, Assistant Dean of Medicine at Brown University School of Medicine. He wrote:

> The case was that of an 81-year-old widow with a traumatic ulcer of the leg. The student-doctor was explaining to the actress-patient her need for near absolute bed rest. This raised the subject of dependency

which was upsetting to the patient, who prided herself on her fierce independence.

Reviewing the videotape of the encounter, it became apparent at a point of great emotional intensity that the student wished to reach out in a gesture of empathy and consolation, but he withdrew.

The videotape was interrupted, and the student was asked what his feelings were at the moment. He said he had wanted to touch the patient but wasn't sure if that was appropriate. We asked the actress to tell what the "patient" was feeling. She replied that she felt very much in need of warmth and human support. Nothing would have been better than having the doctor hold her hand for a few moments. The student's hesitation and reluctance was due to his own uncertainty about what was appropriate in the practice of medicine. Never before in his training had he been told that it was okay to touch patients; for nondiagnostic purposes. By hearing from the "patient" that this would have been a welcome touch and from his instructors that this was not only okay but desirable, a new horizon was opened for this student.[1]

Of course there is appropriate and inappropriate touching, but to be in a position where one feels so unimportant and worthless that one is not worth touching is destructive to the human psyche.

When, through the media, the plight of the untouchables is made known, the response is often overwhelming, testifying to the caring nature of our people. But because the plight of elders is so broad and so unfocused, the standard societal reaction tends to be that of distancing. The responsibility for finding and looking after outcasts rests on a handful of devoted caregivers in mental health, social services, nursing, and welfare groups augmented at times by the police. These are the people who care for those who somehow drop through the cracks in our health-care system.

There is another implication deserving of mention in the no-touch attitude. It is the subtle assumption that elders have lost the need for and interest in physical closeness. Some years ago, a gerontological poster pictured two elders in what was clearly a deep, intimate kiss that suggested sexual overtones. I thought it was a great picture. But there were those who labeled it "disgusting." If old people must be kissed, they are given a peck on the cheek or the forehead and, in some rare occasions, on the lips. Warm intimate kissing is what young people do as seen in late night television shows. In other words, becoming an untouchable elder is the equivalent of becoming asexual. Of course this is nonsense. I find it interesting that my gerontological students experience difficulty in imagining sexual relationships between their parents. They have even greater difficulty in imaging sexual intimacy between their grandparents.

Some years ago, I met with resident managers of church-related homes for elders. I will share only two of their stories. In the first, a middle-aged lady, superintendent of a retirement facility, was showing an elderly couple (prospective residents) the rooms they would be occupying. In the bedroom were two single beds. The woman said, "We want a double bed. I have slept next to this man for the past fifty years and I am not going to stop now." The superintendent sniffed and said, "I would have thought you would be past all that nonsense!"

In the other account, the manager of a large Christian retirement complex hired a young man to do some of the manual work around the institution. The youth was a pleasant fellow, slightly retarded but strongly recommended by a local church group as a reliable worker. The new worker seemed to get along well with everyone. Then the manager began to get complaints from a few of the elderly ladies. One said she had been frightened when she found him standing in the linen closet on her floor. Another said she saw him trying the door of the room of one of the occupants. So the manager fired the young fellow. "Then," he said, "the complaints really came in." Dozens of residents resented the firing. They dismissed the complaints against the young fellow as nonsense. The manager then discovered, to use his words, "that the young man was servicing these elderly ladies and they thought he was great!"

The point I am making is this: *we do not lose our need for touch and warmth and caring as we age. Nor do we lose the ability to enjoy sexual intimacy. These notions, whether they are conveyed in medical training or moral education, are without foundation in fact.*

The danger in classifying elders as untouchables or unimportant in modern society lies in the potential for viewing them as disposable. Some of us cannot forget what happened in Nazi Germany some forty years ago. There, a pattern developed of treating some humans as useless. The first attacks were on the mentally impaired; it was pointed out that these persons made no contribution to society, drained resources, and were therefore disposable. These confused, dependent, helpless German citizens could not defend themselves. Voices of protest went unheeded. Then the classification of disposable humans was extended to include the feeble elderly, the Gypsies, the Jews, and then any other group that the Nazis singled out until some thirteen million were killed.

Could this happen in America? Listen to the voices of those impatient of elders who remain on the job while the young wait for them to retire. Listen to the complaints about medical costs. Listen to the broad hints that triage is already being practiced in Britain and perhaps also in Canada where decisions are made not to treat certain elders.

Moreover, although this is a great and wonderful democracy, there are bigots among us who are intolerant of those representing different ethnic, racial, sexual, and religious orientations. In the United States organized bigots like the Aryan Brotherhood attack blacks and Jews, Hispanics and homosexuals. The potential for age discrimination is always with us. The ethical principle of beneficence requires that the rights of elders be respected and that constant surveillance be mounted to safeguard these rights. The principles on which we act today will be those that govern the baby-boomers when they become elders, when the costs of eldercare may well be tripled, and when there will be more elders than ever before in human history.

It is important to remember that every resident makes some contribution to the development of the nation. It does not really matter whether that contribution was made in the context of some titled or high-sounding service. Everyone counts. Contributions to health and social well-being include more than the work of doctors, nurses, social workers, or researchers. Our health services include the provision of clean working environments, clean streets, and clean neighborhoods so that everyone from dishwashers, through janitors, to street cleaners and garbage disposal teams are important. Each contributes to sanitation and health. Therefore by virtue of being here, no matter how lowly or humble the social status or education or service, elders have earned the right to a dignified old age. Any failure to provide elders with human dignity, food, housing, and health care is to deny our humanity its fullest expression.

The ethical principle is one found in all moral codes and major religious faiths. It is to treat each person as a priceless, one-of-a-kind being, who is never to be replicated in all of human history; who is absolutely unique with a personal DNA structure and genetic heritage; who has experiences and interpretations of experiences that belong to him or her alone; and who is a living library of thoughts, emotions, and concepts.

It is true that some of these living libraries get a bit tattered around the edges. Some hold very ugly and disturbing records of human behavior, but they, too, are part of the human story. There have always been those who must be sheltered or locked away for their own or others' safety. I am not trying to glamorize humanity. The ethical principle is a general one: each individual is unique and precious and deserves to be treated as such.

My third ethical concern relates to elder abuse. The vulnerability of some of the aged makes them targets for scam artists, some of whom are very sophisticated. A widow who received a hefty insurance pay-out on her husband's death was approached by the president of the small religious college from which her husband had graduated. She was informed that it was her duty to use a substantial part of that money to provide scholarships in the dead man's name. Fortunately, she was wise enough to say that she was very distraught over the death and had not had time to work her way through her finances. The gift they recommended would have severely effected her security. Such behavior is unethical. To approach someone who is grieving, in full knowledge that her defenses would be lowered, is utterly reprehensible. This woman was fortunate, she was able to protect herself because she put them off until she could work through her grief.

Perhaps the worst scams are those televangelists who urge listeners to send money with the promise of blessings or of magical healing from illness. I chair a committee that has investigated some of the so-called healers. In one televised program, the evangelist urged those attending his meeting to get rid of their medications in the assurance that Dr. Jesus would heal them. Some members of his audience, including elders, came to the front of the auditorium and threw bottles of pills on the stage. Our investigators gathered the bottles after the service and found nitro-glycerin tablets and other heart medications, oral insulin, digitalis, and so on—life-sustaining medications that this unscrupulous person urged them to discard. By demonstrating his deceptive and unethical techniques, he was forced off the air. But there are others who make fantastic healing claims in the name of religion and who prey on the gullible, including the elderly.

What is more frightening is the increase in the number of reported elder abuse cases that involve physical abuse, including rape, beating, imprisonment, deprivation, starvation, and neglect in addition to financial and psychological abuse. Society is learning to its dismay that we are truly a violent people. In the 1960s and 1970s, the increasing number of reported cases of child abuse and spousal abuse triggered responses that provided laws and agencies to protect children and battered wives. During the 1980s, attention was focused on elder abuse, particularly on treatment in nursing homes. There can be no question that in some poorly managed nursing homes, helpless elders have been severely abused. Horror stories, complete with pictures of elders with raw bed sores, lying in feces or on urine-soaked sheets, held in place by straps, doped with drugs to keep them quiet, have aroused public anger and have resulted in investigations and reforms.

But most of the abuse is familial. The victim is often a woman over the age of seventy-five who is physically or mentally dependent. The typical abuser is a relative, often a child of the victim. At times the abuse reflects familial patterns of violence that have become the customary ways of settling disputes or problems within the family. Sometimes there is an element of revenge. One folk rhyme reads:

> When I was a laddie, I lived with my granny,
> And many a beating my granny did give me.
> Now I'm a man and I live with my granny
> And I do to my granny what she did to me.

The horror stories reporting familial abuse surpass those of nursing homes and range from cruel, cutting, and debasing remarks to distortions of facts that lead to near madness; from physical beatings that bruise, scar, and break bones, to neglect, starvation, and denial of medicines and medical treatment; from imprisonment with restraints, often in dark, filthy, infested rooms or attics, to theft and misuse of elder finances. Some abuse even results in the elder's death. The brutality is not restricted to any racial, religious, or ethnic group and is practiced among the wealthy as often as among the poor. Like dependent children and spouses, some elders have become targets for violence and deprivation. The number of reported cases of elder abuse mounts steadily and it is estimated that many instances of maltreatment go unreported.

Why don't elders call for help? Some do so when they learn that their complaints will be heard. Others refrain because they have been told that no one will believe them. Some have been persuaded that somehow they are at fault and deserve maltreatment. Others hesitate out of pride, feeling that reporting will cast a shadow on the reputation of the family and on themselves as inadequte parents. Still others have been terrorized into believing that should they make a report, the abuser will increase the abuse. Many are in a helpless situation and unable to make their condition known.

The ethical issue is obvious. *No one has the right or should have the freedom to abuse another person verbally, psychologically, financially, physically, or spiritually. Abuse in any form should not be tolerated, whether it is done in the name of religion or some school of psychology or education. No one should be subjected to abuse by government representatives, institutional personnel, or family members. Our ethical stance must be that of zero tolerance of any form of abuse.* Abuse must be reported and dealt with by removing victims into protective custody for treatment of wounds—whether they be physical, psychological, or spiritual—and by taking abusers into custody where they cannot reach victims and where they receive remedial counseling or appropriate legal punishment.

My fourth ethical point relates to the question of *meaning in life.* The search for meaning is an issue that confronts every thoughtful person who is not willing to accept simplistic answers or dogma. As my students put the question: "What's it all about?" My answer is always the same, "I don't know," because it would be pompous and foolish of me or anyone else to try to respond with a statement concerning the ultimate meaning of human existence. Philosophers and theologians have wrestled with the question for ages. What we *can* understand is how individuals give meaning to their present existence.

Meaning is found in different ways. If one is part of an extended family with deep bonding patterns, meaning may be found in family relationships. A mother finds meaning in being the best mother and wife she can be; a father, in being the best father and husband he can be; a son, in being the best son and brother and later the best father he can be; and a daughter, in fulfilling her role as daughter, sister, then perhaps wife and mother to her own family.

Some find meaning in work. I have been with engineers and carpenters and bricklayers who point with pride to what they have helped bring into being, whether it be a high-rise building, a piece of home furniture, or a noise barrier on a freeway. I have met gardeners, seamstresses, cooks, and homemakers, each of whom delights in what he or she has created.

Some find meaning in a faith system that links them to an afterlife or to reincarnation. What they do in this life has meaning for the next.

Sometimes, however, what we count on to bring meaning undergoes change, and with time it fails us. Some become so enmeshed in their work that when their working days are passed they do not know how to retire. They have never learned to pause and enjoy other dimensions of life. Some, out of sheer boredom, retreat into senility. Some become crotchety, complaining grumps who seem to do nothing but get on other people's nerves. These individuals feel they have outlived their usefulness. Their present existence has no significance. They retreat from life, or declare their presence with a vengeance by criticizing everyone and everything.

We are in a migratory age. Families separate and move to different parts of the state, the nation, and even the world. When families gather for festal occasions or vacations, sometimes the old intimacy has gone. Each family has developed its own life patterns. The elders who fancied growing old with their families around them feel estranged and abandoned. The family bond does not always give meaning.

In the event that a spouse dies, the remaining elder may be suddenly and completely isolated in retirement. Women, for a variety of reasons, seem to survive the death of a husband better than men do the death of a wife. If the wife dies first, quite often the husband dies within a year.

A colleague, a noted therapist and sociologist, with whom I co-taught courses on death and dying, suffered the loss of his wife after her long illness. He had been a wonderful nurse to her during the final stages of her cancer. After she died, he followed all the healthy steps for griev-

ing and survival that we had been teaching. Suddenly, at the close of
the semester, he was hospitalized. His legs refused to cooperate and he
couldn't walk. Examinations found absolutely nothing physically wrong
with him, but he had to undergo rehabilitation training. His ailment was
psychosomatic. Unlike some grieving husbands, he did not die, but the
physical reaction to his feelings of loss incapacitated him.

Elders who are isolated by death or by distance from significant others
often sense an estrangement from life that induces withdrawal. Such
withdrawal into the self induces depression, reinforces isolation, and moves
the person toward inclusion among the untouchables, those who feel helpless, hopeless, and unlovable. The research by Martin Seligman has pointed
to the potential for serious physical reactions and even death as the elderly
react to feelings of helplessness. He has pointed out that elders in institutionalized settings can become depressed and helpless as they feel their
control over life diminishing. He writes:

> Institutionalized patients, whether in terminal cancer wards, leukemic
> children's wards, or old-age homes, should be given maximum control
> over all aspects of their daily lives: choice of omelets or scrambled eggs
> for breakfast, blue or red curtains, going to the movies on Wednesdays
> or Thursdays, whether they wake or sleep late. If the theory of helpless-
> ness set forth here has any validity, these people may live longer, may
> show more spontaneous remissions, and will certainly be much happier.[2]

The ethical principle is simple. We all need to feel important. We
all need to feel in control. We all need to belong and to know that we
are significant members of the human family. We need to know that our
choices are heeded and that we matter. Because we are all so hungry
for recognition, it takes very little effort to acknowledge the presence of
others, to speak a word of greeting, to tell someone he or she looks nice
when that is true, or to compliment someone for efforts made. I am not
suggesting that we take on a simplistic Pollyanna attitude in which nothing but the good and positive are found in every situation. What I am
calling for is the recognition of the personhood of others. Perhaps the
telephone company has it right with their "reach out and touch someone" slogan.

My final ethical issue focuses on *freedom of choice, the very sensitive issue of euthanasia, and the individual's right to choose to die with
dignity*. There can only be praise for the marvelous advances in medical
and health sciences that have helped to extend the anticipated life span
from forty-seven at the turn of the century to the mid to late seventies
as it is today. Diseases that once ravaged families have been brought under

control with modern medical treatment and preventive vaccination; we are much more inclined to emphasize diet and exercise; and medical science continues to expand the numbers of those who live into old age.

But extended life does not guarantee meaningful, satisfactory, or dignified existence. Some who have contracted incurable diseases, such as certain forms of cancer, have been kept alive against their will by machines, gastrol feeding tubes, and intravenous medication. In some instances, even without the employment of heroic measures to sustain life, the individual continued to live, often in pain that could only be controlled by medications that produce a semi-coma state.

The development of the hospice concept has provided aid for terminally ill persons and their families. Hospice workers consult, meet with, and work with the dying person and his or her loved ones. No attempts are made to treat the incurable disease. Pain control under the patient's management enables some terminally ill persons to remain at home. In other instances, where facilities are available, the dying person can be at peace in the relaxed and caring atmosphere of the hospice. The aim is to provide an atmosphere in which the patient can die with dignity, without intubation, without machines, and without medical efforts to sustain life.

Living wills provide individuals with the opportunity to express their personal wishes for treatment should they become incapacitated with a terminal illness or a life-threatening condition. This will—executed and witnessed while the person is of sound mind and body, with copies given to family members, attorneys, doctors, and hospital personnel—can provide for the removal of life-support systems in the event that the person facing imminent death experiences intractable pain or perhaps lapses into an irreversible coma. In such cases the doctor may act, knowing that the patient has sanctioned the act. Presently, the living will has legal status in thirty-seven states in America, which means that doctors can act in accordance with patients' wishes without fear of prosecution by someone who disagrees with such life-terminating decisions.

A second document, the Durable Power of Attorney for Health Care, provides that should a person be in a terminal condition and unable to make his or her wishes known, perhaps due to coma, an appointed person may act on behalf of the patient and call for the cessation of heroic treatment.

Both the living will and the Durable Power of Attorney for Health Care are designed to permit the terminally ill patient to express the choice to die through the removal of life-support equipment and the cessation of medicinal treatment. This form of euthanasia is known as *passive euthanasia*. However, as the world learned in the Karen Ann Quinlan case, removal of life-support equipment does not necessarily bring death. Karen

Ann lived for years in irreversible coma after the breathing apparatus was removed. Her lower brain stem kept her heart beating and her lungs working.[3]

Now efforts are under way to legalize *active euthanasia,* by which a medical doctor, at the request of a terminally ill patient, may administer a lethal drug and cause death. Today, such procedures are accepted only in Holland. Elsewhere, whenever such acts are performed, the doctor, or anyone else who performs the act, faces homicide charges if the deed becomes known. There are serious ethical problems involved that have to do with control over one's own death and with the quality of life for terminally ill patients, some of whom writhe in pain that cannot be properly controlled.

Let me illustrate the problem. A few years ago, I received a phone call from a Canadian university professor. Her mother was in agony in the final stages of invasive cancer. Medications left her groggy and only partially controlled the pain. She begged her daughter to do something to help her die. The daughter asked me, "What can I do?"

How could I respond to such a request from a person I had never met and who was several thousand miles away? Yet how could I dismiss this *crie de couer?* I asked for more details, got the daughter's address, the phone number of the hospital room, and so on. Then I said, "Talk to your doctor."

The next few days were difficult for me as I reflected on the daughter's and the mother's plight. Finally, I dialed the hospital room and the daughter answered and said, "I am so glad you phoned. I have just given my mother the lethal injection." She had done as I had suggested and that day the doctor had put a syringe in her hand saying, "I never want to talk to you again about this." He then walked away.

The professor and her mother said their last farewells and expressed their love for one another before the lethal injection. The mother died relaxed with a contented smile on her face. Some fifteen months later, the professor and I met in California at a conference. She experienced no guilt for ending her mother's life. Hers was an act of love. In compliance with her mother's wishes, she had shortened the period of suffering that could have gone on for several more weeks. Which was the higher ethical responsibility, to terminate the pain and suffering or to sit by and let her mother suffer and do nothing to help? Which would be the greater act of love?

Euthanasia, both passive and active, will continue to be an important ethical concern for gerontology. Most elders are healthy. Most die peaceful deaths. For the minority who do not and for those whose deaths are marked by protracted suffering, the desire will be to have control over the ending of life. For these persons, to be kept alive by medical machinery, or to die slowly in agonizing pain, is not to die with dignity. They desire to be in control with the power to choose.

CONCLUSION

Aging in these final years of the twentieth century continues to present us with increasingly complex ethical choices. Some terrible things have happened to elders, perhaps things that had been happening for centuries but which have never surfaced in the ways they have today. There are also some wonderful things happening. Can we produce ethical guidelines that will help do the greatest good for the greatest number and at the same time enable individuals to feel in control of their destiny and to live and die with dignity and with feelings of self-respect?

Ethical leadership in eldercare calls for a balance between utilitarianism and individualism. The challenge is dramatic because we deal with a multi-dimensional unity and a multiplicity of individual identities: a unity of connectedness by virtue of being elders in a nation, and a diversity developed out of national pluralism that encourages unique identity. This calls for the development of responses to eldercare that recognize the unique and definitive worth of each individual without weighing the person's health status or usefulness to society.

As we seek to maximize benefits and extend the length and quality of life, the greatest controversies are going to be over costs. America is not a poor nation, but it may be necessary to rethink the distribution of national wealth, possibly by increasing taxes. But what are the alternatives? As the number of elders increases, what kind of national ethic will be developed? Will it be an ethic that subtly undermines confidence in the ability of the national system to provide for its citizens so that they will look with fear and uncertainty to their old age? Do we simply extend working years so that the work ethic will be dominant and then judge or reward elders on the basis of how long they can work and contribute to the gross national product? Will we develop policies that deny the best treatment to elders simply because they are old? What kind of a national ethical formula can we develop to inspire us to live according to the highest value system?

There is need for a vision that recognizes what it has meant to citizens to be free in an open, democratic society—a vision that honors the pluralism of concepts, religions, and races and does not practice bigotry based on sex, religion, race, or age. The bringing about of that society is the task that engages all of us. Young people need to feel secure as they look ahead to old age, but that can happen only by positively influencing the ways in which the aged are treated today. We dare not support a human discard philosophy that confines useful, wise, and sensitive humans to the waste heap solely on the basis of age.

We seek to develop laws and codes to guide us in our responses to human need. When such codes embrace the highest and noblest ethical principles, they provide guidance for responses that recognize the worth of the individual. When such ethical standards become internalized by those who administer the regulations, they build character. People of high ethical standing will seek to act for the greatest benefit of individual elders. Can we develop ethical statements relating to individuals and to institutions? I think we can.

It is the ethical responsibility of the elder, indeed the responsibility of every citizen, to act and live so as to bring out the best in oneself and the best in others, to call forth the highest and noblest response in ourselves and in others so that each of us contributes to the betterment of the future of our children, grandchildren, and great-grandchildren. In other words, the ethical individual lives to move the world a tiny bit closer to the highest dreams and visions of our greatest thinkers, religionists, philosophers, psychologists, poets, and visionaries.

The ethical stance of institutions and government should be to create an environment in which individuals can maximize their growth and attain their highest goals. It is the responsibility of institutions, including the government and those empowered to act by the people, to seek to preserve the dignity and self-worth of elders. This ethic calls for the setting of high goals and working toward them. It calls for challenging unacceptable behavior in anyone who comes in contact with elders. It means an unwillingness to give up on a problem or on a person, no matter how difficult the challenge may be. It means recognition that freedom, as part of the national ethos, has encouraged and produced individual differences that deserve respect.

We who are advocates for elders must go out as teachers, holding up the ethical ideal as the human ideal, as the ideal for all, embracing all, binding on all. It is the ideal of a society in which no elder, indeed, no man or woman and no class of men and women, shall be used as tools for the lusts of others, for the ambitions of others, for the greed of others, or as targets for the anger of others. It is the ideal of a society in which every human life, whether young or old, shall be esteemed and treated as a sacred utterance of the universe.[4] This is our challenge. This is our commission. If we take it seriously, then we can face the future, with its growing numbers of elders, in the confidence that both we and they will be treated with dignity, respect, and care.

NOTES

1. Helen Colton, *The Gift of Touch* (New York: Seaview/Putnam, 1983), p. 118.

2. Martin E. P. Seligman, *Helplessness* (San Francisco: W. H. Freeman and Co., 1975), p. 183.

3. Perhaps the best-known case of partial brain death is that of Karen Ann Quinlan, a twenty-one-year-old woman, who lapsed into a coma on April 14, 1975. She had been on a crash diet and without having eaten all day attended a party where she drank a few gin-and-tonics and later took aspirin and a therapeutic dose of tranquilizer. Shortly afterward she lapsed into a coma, the true cause of which was never determined inasmuch as the drugs and alcohol were deemed insufficient causes. Within a month, her body had shrunk to a mere seventy pounds and was contorted into a gross simulation of the fetal position. Her life was sustained by machines that pumped air into her lungs and tubes that delivered food and antibiotics into her system. Neurologists determined that she had entered into a rigid, irreversible vegetative state and that her cognitive brain functions had ceased. Only the parts of the brain controlling her breathing, facial movement, blood pressure and heart rate, and to some degree her body temperature were still functioning. It was clear that Karen would never recover the use of her brain and that her twisted limbs would never untwine. She was, medically speaking, "brain dead"; she would never be cognitively aware.

On July 31, her parents requested that the respirator be removed and that Karen be permitted to die. The hospital authorities and the doctor, although sympathetic, refused inasmuch as Karen was of age. And since her parents were not her guardians, they could not authorize the removal of the respirator—only Karen could do that, and she was in coma. The lower courts upheld the decision, but on March 31, 1976, the Supreme Court of New Jersey reversed the decision and established the first right-to-die ruling in legal history. Despite the Supreme Court ruling, the hospital and physician in charge did not drastically alter their treatment—indeed, in May, a temperature control device was added as a technological support. On May 17th, all support machines were removed, but Karen continued to live, breathing on her own. Her life and death were now under the control of her own body, augmented of course by hospital care and feeding. She died in 1985.

4. This statement is drawn in part from Felix Adler, *Life and Destiny* (New York: McLure, Phillips & Co., 1903), pp. 140–41.

Contributors

TED BALL is president of PoliCorp., a political and corporate relations company specializing in public-affairs analysis, strategic-communications planning, and government-affairs management.

MARY ANN BARNHART is a licensed professional counselor and currently a geriatric therapist at Denton Regional Medical Center, Pathways Psychiatric Program, Denton, Texas.

RICH BAYLY is the executive director of the Alberta Long-Term Care Association.

LEAH BUTURAIN is a consultant to Community Based Services for the Elderly in California.

JOY CALKIN is associate vice-president (academic) at the University of Calgary.

RUSSELL CARR is an associate with William M. Mercer, Ltd., an international consulting firm specializing in human resources and organizational strategy. He heads the public policy and management practice in the firm's Edmonton, Alberta, office.

GERALD A. LARUE is emeritus professor of religion at the University of Southern California, Los Angeles. He is also adjunct professor of gerontology at the university's Andrus Center.

PETER N. MCCRACKEN is clinical head of the Department of Geriatric Medicine at Edmonton General Hospital, Edmonton, Alberta.

MARK NOVAK is associate dean (academic) of the Continuing Education Division at the University of Manitoba.

MICHAEL RACHLIS, M.D. (FRCP) is an author and a private consultant in health policy.

EVA SKINNER is a member of the board of directors of the American Association of Retired Persons.

FERNANDO M. TORRES-GIL is professor in the Department of Social Welfare, University of California, Los Angeles, and president of the American Society on Aging.

MONIQUE VÉZINA is Canada's minister of state for seniors.

KATHLEEN H. WILBUR is assistant professor and senior research associate at the Andrus Center, University of Southern California, Los Angeles.

LINDA A. WRAY is a research associate at the Andrus Center, University of Southern California, Los Angeles.